Color Atlas of
Basic Histology

A LANGE MEDICAL BOOK

Irwin Berman, PhD
Associate Professor of Cell Biology and Anatomy
University of Miami School of Medicine
Miami, Florida

APPLETON & LANGE
Norwalk, Connecticut

Copyright © 1993 by Appleton & Lange
Simon & Schuster Business and Professional Group

93 94 95 96 97 / 10 9 8 7 6 5 4 3 2 1

Prentice Hall International (UK) Limited, *London*
Prentice Hall of Australia Pty. Limited, *Sydney*
Prentice Hall Canada, Inc., *Toronto*
Prentice Hall Hispanoamericana, S.A., *Mexico*
Prentice Hall of India Private Limited, *New Delhi*
Prentice Hall of Japan, Inc., *Tokyo*
Simon & Schuster Asia Pte. Ltd., *Singapore*
Editora Prentice Hall do Brasil Ltda., *Rio de Janeiro*
Prentice Hall, *Englewood Cliffs, New Jersey*

Library of Congress Cataloging-in-Publication Data
Berman, Irwin, 1924–
    Color atlas of basic histology / Irwin Berman.
        p.   cm.
    ISBN 0-8385-0445-0
    1. Histology—Atlases. I. Title
    [DNLM: 1. Histology—atlases. QS 517 B516c]
QM557.B425   1993
611'.018'0222—dc20
DNLM/DLC
for Library of Congress   92-48796
                                                           CIP

On the cover is a photomicrograph of an osteoclast (Fig. 4-10). Courtesy of Mr. Ralph Alvarez.

Cover design by Penny Kindzierski
Acquisitions Editor: John Dolan
Production Editor: Karen Davis
Production Services: Peter Strupp/Princeton Editorial Associates
Designer: Janice Barsevich Bielawa

PRINTED IN THE UNITED STATES OF AMERICA

Contents

Preface

The purpose of this atlas is to provide students with a simple, concise, readily accessible source of morphologic information for use in the identification of tissues and organs in histology laboratories. The atlas can also serve as an independent study and review resource. As the underlying principle of this atlas is simple presentation of the essential imagery of microscopic anatomy, it is offered as a supplement to lecture and text material, not a substitute for it.

The atlas is a compendium primarily of color pictures taken at the light microscope level (some scanning and electron micrographs are included) that have been selected for the clarity with which they depict the basic morphologic characteristics of tissues and organs that students need to be able to recognize. The subject matter is presented in oversized photomicrographs. Labeling of photomicrographs has been kept as simple as possible, guiding students directly to the key morphologic features that identify the subject and to structures that are important in understanding the function of the subject. The photomicrographs, unless stated otherwise, were taken from human material stained with hematoxylin and eosin, the dyes most commonly used in histology and pathology. The tissue source for the electron micrographs is also noted. For the organ systems, wherever possible, a flow of morphologic information from low- to high-magnification images is presented. The magnification of each image is a final figure taking into account photomicrographic and print magnifications.

Since the identification of bone marrow cells is a difficult exercise in histology, a concise description of the major morphologic changes which occur during development of the erythroid and myeloid cell series accompanies the photomicrographs in Chapter 9, "The Identification of Bone Marrow Cells."

Acknowledgments

It is a pleasure for me to acknowledge and thank the following individuals who so willingly and generously contributed to this atlas: Mr. Ralph Alvarez, Dr. Mary Bartlett Bunge, Mr. Jean-Pierre Brunschwig, Dr. Ronald G. Clark, Ms. Susan J. Decker, Dr. Joanne M. Howard, Dr. Douglas R. Kelly, Mr. Andrew Lee, Dr. Jacques Padawer, Dr. Melanie M. Pratt, Dr. Mikel H. Snow, Dr. Gary E. Wise, and Dr. Richard L. Wood.

My thanks to Mr. John J. Dolan, Medical Editor, and Ms. Karen W. Davis, Production Supervisor, for their enthusiasm for the project, for their many helpful suggestions, and for making the publication process an informative and pleasurable experience. I also wish to thank Ms. Ruth W. Weinberg, formerly of Appleton & Lange, who originally presented my proposal for a color atlas of histology to the editorial board of Appleton & Lange and was its first sponsoring editor.

I express my deep appreciation to Mr. Gilbert S. Kahn and the Janet A. Hooker Charitable Trust, whose gifts helped defray the cost of photographic supplies, film processing, and making of print proofs.

Color Atlas of
Basic Histology

A LANGE MEDICAL BOOK

1 Epithelial Tissue

FIGURE 1-1

Simple squamous epithelium (arrows) of the serosa of the small intestine. This epithelium is also referred to as mesothelium. × 344.

FIGURE 1-2

En face view of the simple squamous epithelium of the peritoneum. Note the very close association of the lateral cell boundaries of adjoining cells. × 869.

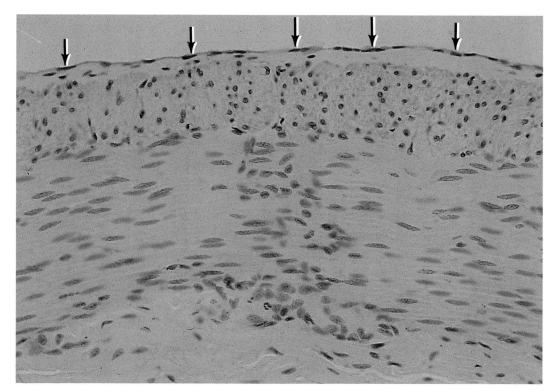

figure 1-1

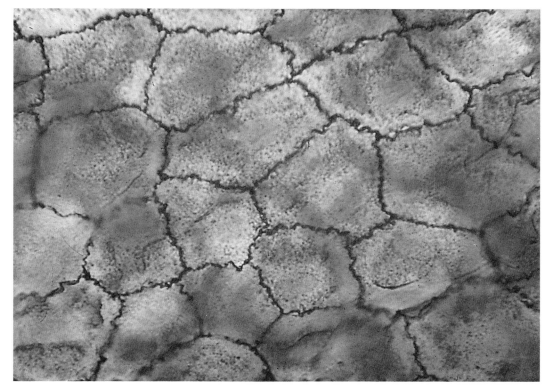

figure 1-2

FIGURE 1-3
Simple squamous epithelial cells (arrows) which line the lumen of blood vessels. This epithelium is also referred to as endothelium. × 869.

FIGURE 1-4
Simple squamous epithelial cells (arrows) from the parietal layer of Bowman's capsule in a renal corpuscle. × 140.

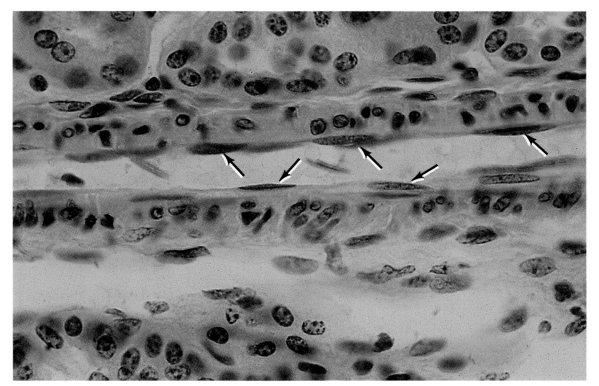

figure 1-3

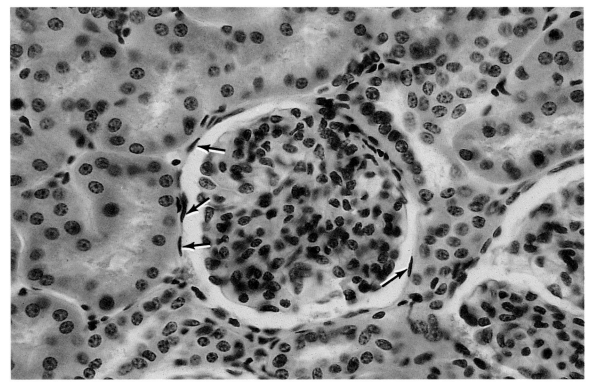

figure 1-4

FIGURE 1-5
Cuboidal epithelium of kidney collecting tubules in longitudinal and cross section (arrow). × 344.

FIGURE 1-6
Cross section of the cuboidal epithelium of thyroid follicles. Note that in both cross and longitudinal sections, cuboidal cell height and width are approximately equal. × 344.

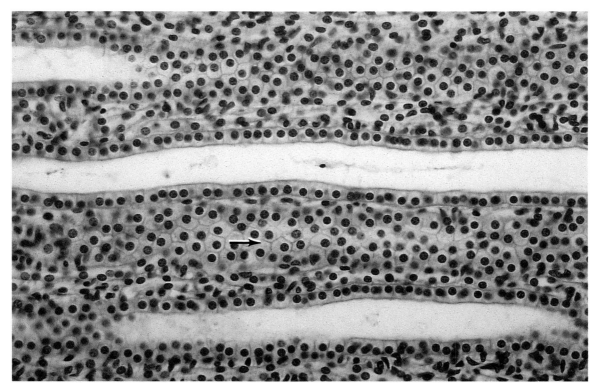

figure 1-5

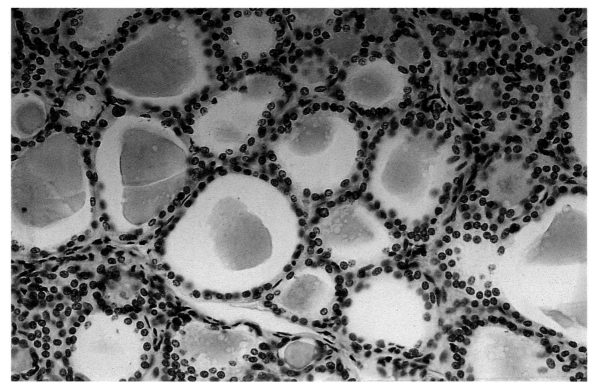

figure 1-6

FIGURE 1-7
Cross section of the cuboidal epithelium of the proximal convoluted tubules of the kidney. The microvillus (brush) border of these cells is not well preserved in fixation, which accounts for the fuzzy pinkish material within the tubule's lumen. × 344.

FIGURE 1-8
Simple columnar epithelium of the gall bladder. The space between some cells is an artifact of slide preparation. Note the difference between the height and width of the cells and the basal location of nuclei in this type of epithelium. × 344.

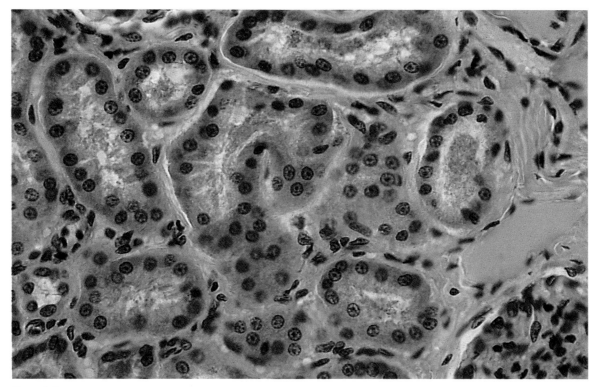

figure 1-7

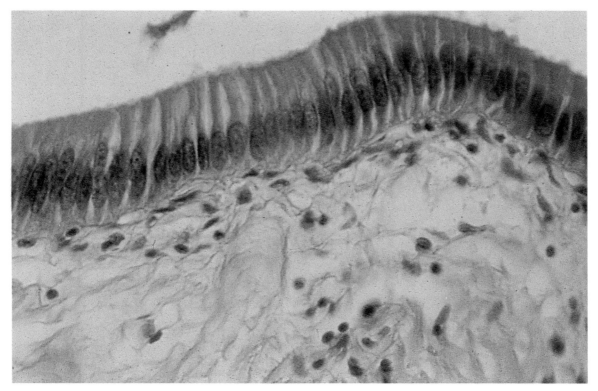

figure 1-8

FIGURE 1-9
Simple columnar epithelium of a kidney collecting duct resting on a thin basement membrane (arrows). × 560.

FIGURE 1-10
Simple columnar epithelium with goblet cells (arrows) of the ileum. × 344.

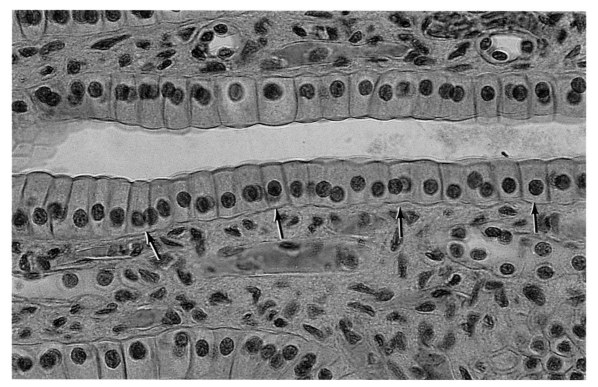

figure 1-9

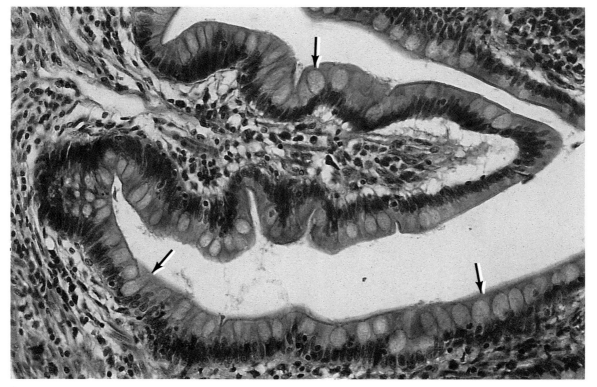

figure 1-10

FIGURE 1-11
Pseudostratified columnar ciliated (arrows) epithelium of the trachea. Monkey; × 560.

FIGURE 1-12
Nonkeratinized stratified squamous epithelium of the esophagus. Monkey; × 344.

FIGURE 1-13
Stratified squamous keratinized (arrows) epithelium of thin skin. × 344.

FIGURE 1-14
Transitional epithelium of the ureter. × 344.

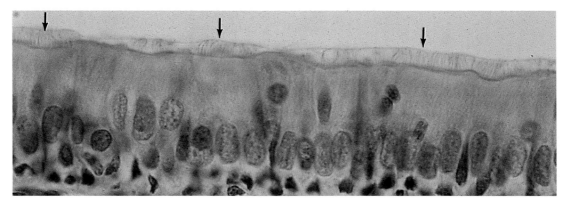

figure 1-11

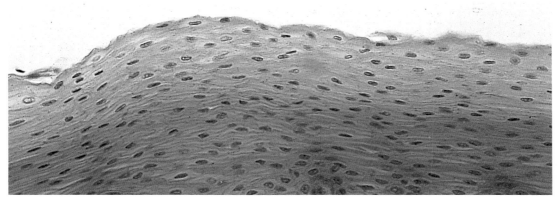

figure 1-12

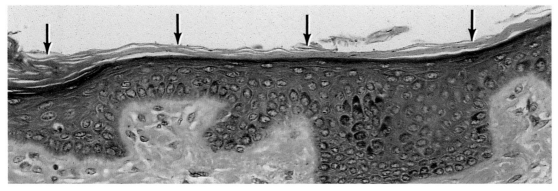

figure 1-13

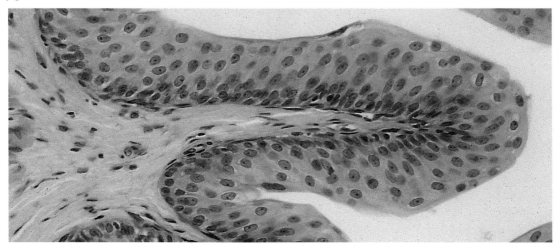

figure 1-14

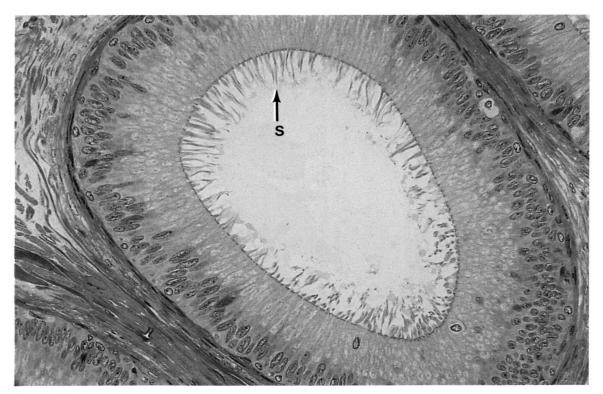

figure 1-15

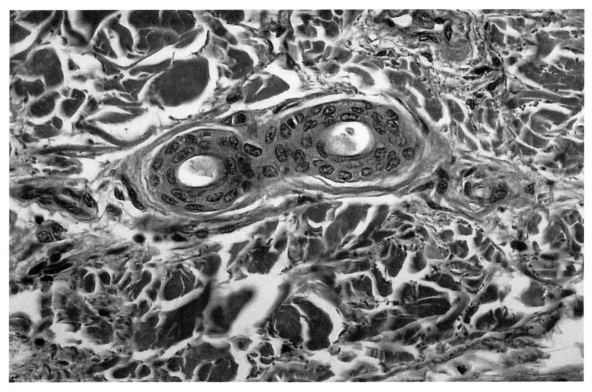

figure 1-16

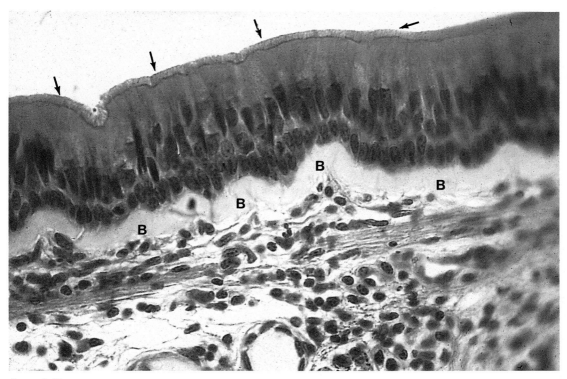

figure 1-17

FIGURE 1-15
Pseudostratified columnar epithelium with stereocilia (S) of the epididymis. Compare the stereocilia with cilia in Figures 1-11 and 1-17. × 344.

FIGURE 1-16
Stratified cuboidal epithelium of a sweat gland duct in skin. × 560.

FIGURE 1-17
Pseudostratified columnar ciliated (arrows) epithelium of the trachea. Note the prominent basement membrane (B). Compare this basement membrane with that in Figure 1-9. × 344.

2 Connective Tissue Proper

FIGURE 2-1
Photomicrograph of mesenchymal connective tissue from embryonic mouse jaw. Note the pleomorphic nature of the mesenchymal cells (arrows) and the amorphous appearance of the ground substance (GS). Masson's stain. × 140.

FIGURE 2-2
Photomicrograph of mucous connective tissue of the umbilical cord. Note the stellate nature of the fibroblasts (arrows) and wispy aggregates of collagen (C). × 140.

FIGURE 2-3
Photomicrograph of loose connective tissue (areolar) from the peritoneum illustrating fibroblasts (F), collagen (C), and elastic fibers (E). A branching blood vessel is seen coursing through the connective tissue. × 344.

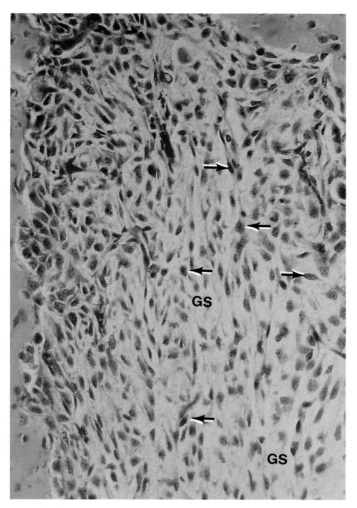

figure 2-1

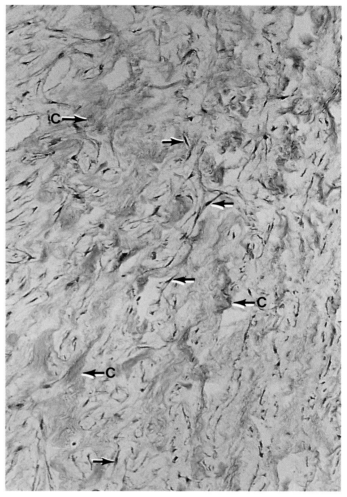

figure 2-2

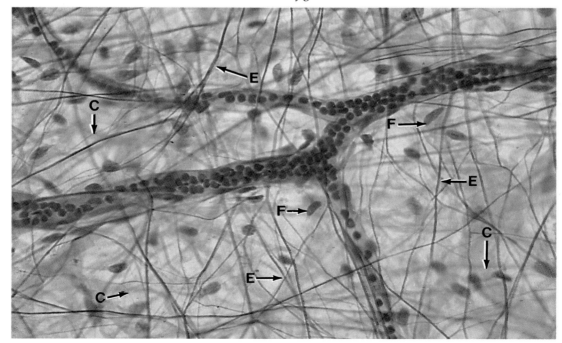

figure 2-3

FIGURE 2-4
Photomicrograph of loose irregular connective tissue (L) of the lamina propria of the esophagus. × 140.

FIGURE 2-5
Photomicrograph illustrating the differing morphologies of loose irregular connective tissue (L), dense irregular connective tissue (D), and skeletal muscle (M). × 140.

FIGURE 2-6
Photomicrograph of fibroblasts (arrows) in loose connective tissue. P, plasma cell; C, collagen. × 869.

FIGURE 2-7
Photomicrograph of fibroblasts (arrows) in dense irregular connective tissue. Note the thick wavy collagen bundles (C) in contrast to those seen in Figure 2-6. × 869.

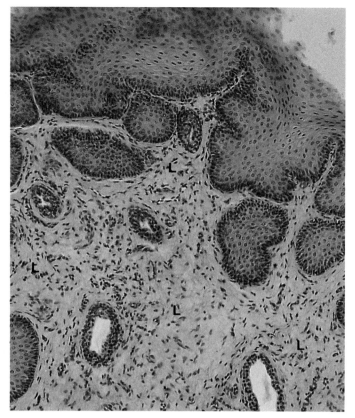

figure 2-4

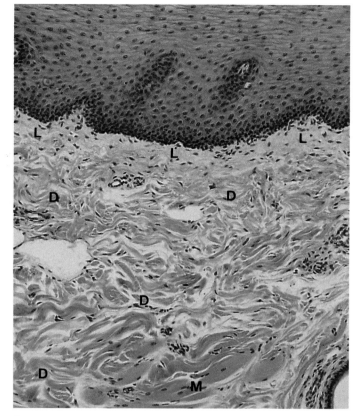

figure 2-5

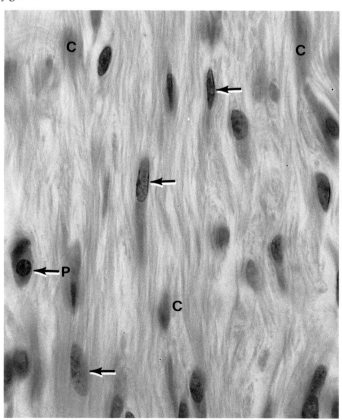

figure 2-6

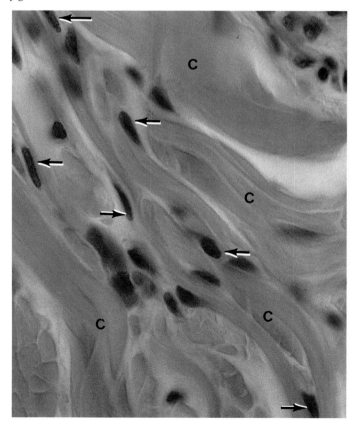

figure 2-7

FIGURE 2-8

Photomicrograph of dense irregular connective tissue. Note the wavy unorientated collagen bundles (C) and fibroblasts (arrows). P, plasma cell. × 344.

FIGURE 2-9

Photomicrograph of dense regular connective tissue. Note the parallel orientation of collagen (C) and fibroblasts (arrows), in contrast to the haphazard arrangement of these elements seen in Figure 2-8. × 344.

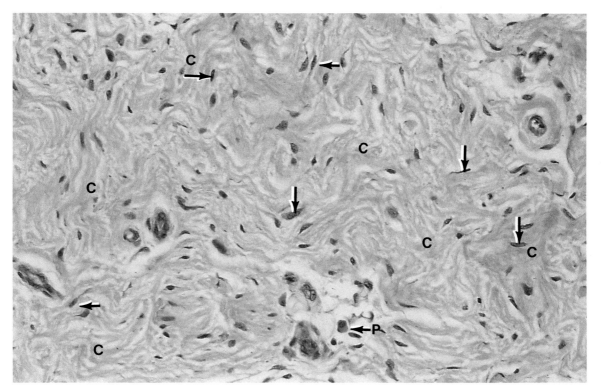

figure 2-8

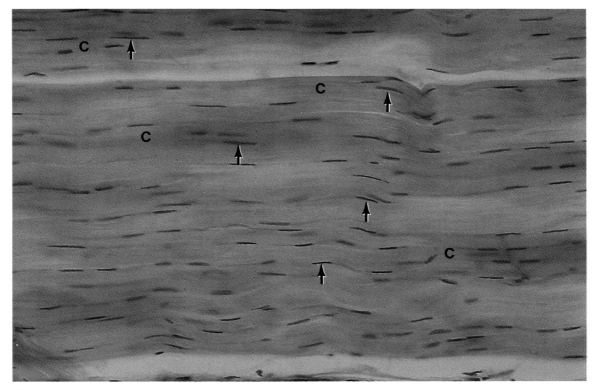

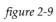

figure 2-9

FIGURE 2-10
Higher-power photomicrograph of a portion of Figure 2-8 illustrating three different cell types found in connective tissue: plasma cells (P), lymphocytes (L), and fibroblasts (F). C, collagen. × 869.

FIGURE 2-11
Electron micrograph of a plasma cell illustrating a well-developed rough endoplasmic reticulum (RE), which characterizes this cell at the ultrastructural level. NP, nucleus of the plasma cell; G, Golgi region. An eosinophil (E) is also depicted. Rat; × 5010.

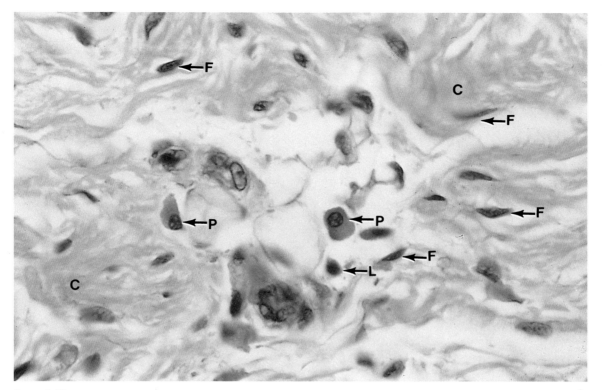

figure 2-10

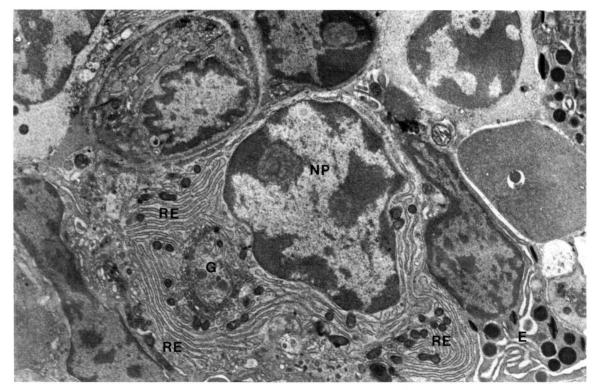

figure 2-11

FIGURE 2-12
Photomicrograph of mast cells (arrows) in connective tissue between skeletal muscle fibers (S) of the tongue. Azure stain. Rat; × 560.

FIGURE 2-13
Photomicrograph of mast cells from a drop preparation of peritoneal fluid. Toluidine blue stain. Mouse; × 5375. (Courtesy of Dr. Jacques Padawer.)

FIGURE 2-14
Radioautograph of mast cells from the peritoneal fluid of a young rat injected with tritiated thymidine. Note the specific localization of silver grains in the nucleus (N) of the labeled cell (L), indicating that fully differentiated mast cells are not postmitotic. UL, unlabeled mast cell. Toluidine blue stain. × 5375. (Courtesy of Dr. Jacques Padawer.)

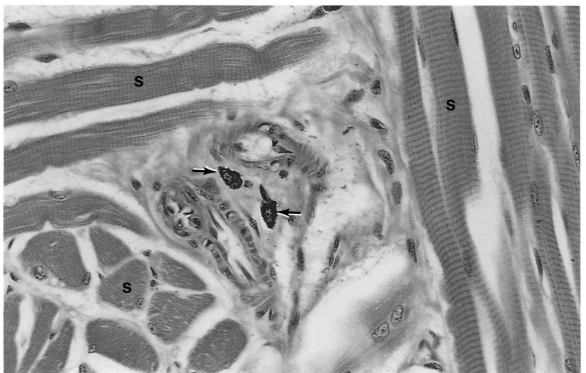

figure 2-12

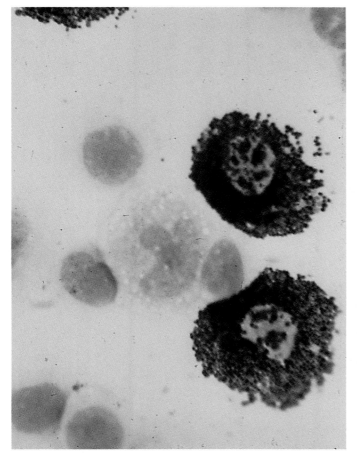

figure 2-13

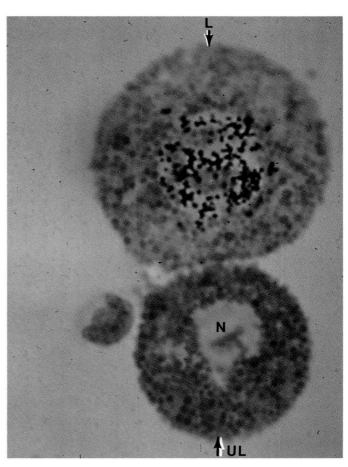

figure 2-14

FIGURE 2-15
Electron micrograph of a mast cell. Note the large electron-dense granules (GR), nucleus (N), Golgi region (G), and mitochondria (arrows). Rat; × 16,086. (Courtesy of Dr. Jacques Padawer.)

FIGURE 2-16
Electron micrograph of a macrophage illustrating secondary lysosomes (S). N, nucleus; M, mitochondria. Rat; × 27,823. (Courtesy of Dr. Jacques Padawer.)

FIGURE 2-17
Electron micrograph of an eosinophil. Note the ovoid granules (arrows) with paracrystalline inclusions which characterize this cell at the ultrastructural level. N, nucleus. Mouse; × 8136.

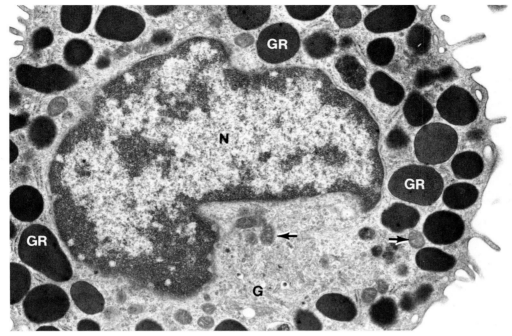

figure 2-15

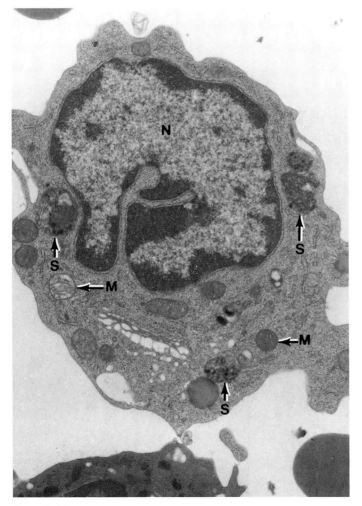

figure 2-16

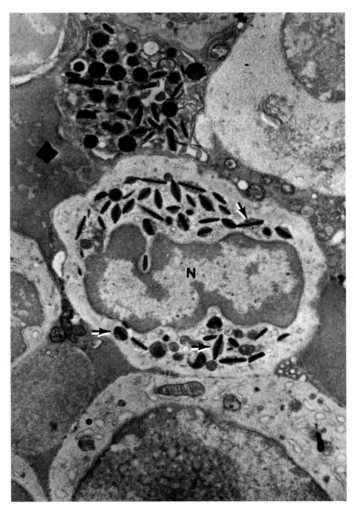

figure 2-17

FIGURE 2-18

Photomicrograph illustrating adipose tissue. The lipid of the unilocular adipose cells (A) is extracted during slide preparation, giving the cells a vacuolated appearance. V, blood vessel; S, skeletal muscle. × 140.

FIGURE 2-19

Photomicrograph of unilocular adipose cells. Note the peripherally located nuclei (arrows) of the adipocytes (A). Lipid was extracted from the cells during slide preparation. S, skeletal muscle. Azure stain. Rat; × 344.

FIGURE 2-20

Photomicrograph of unilocular adipose cells fixed and stained with osmium tetroxide. Note that lipid (L) with this type of fixation is retained by many cells. Adipose cells (A) from which lipid has been completely extracted are apparent. × 344.

FIGURE 2-21

Photomicrograph illustrating unilocular adipose cells after staining with Sudan red, an oil-soluble dye. Note that lipid (L) completely fills the adipose cells. × 560.

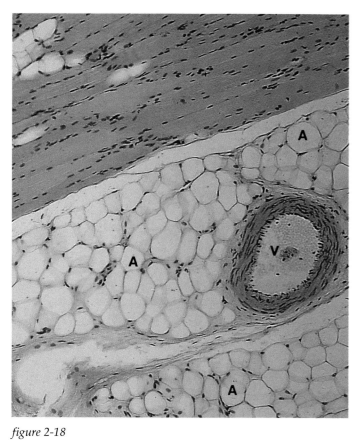

figure 2-18

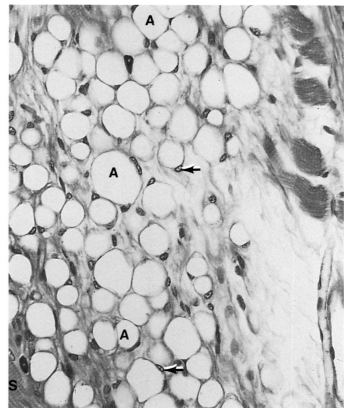

figure 2-19

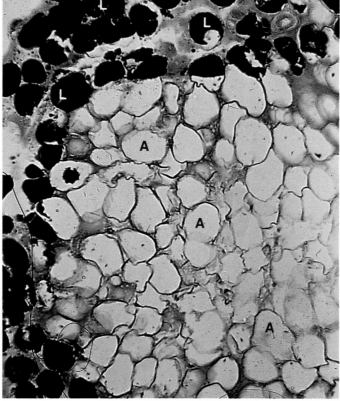

figure 2-20

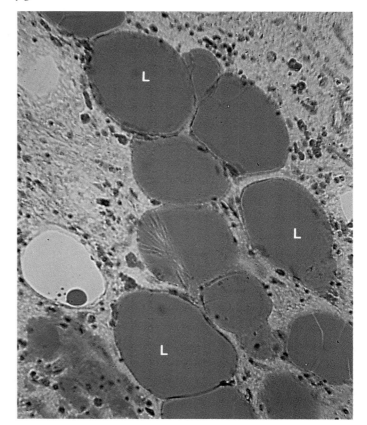

figure 2-21

FIGURE 2-22
Photomicrograph of elastic connective tissue in the tunica media of the aorta. Note the typical wavy appearance of the thick bundles of elastic fibers (arrows). Weigert's stain. × 344.

FIGURE 2-23
Photomicrograph of reticular connective tissue in a lymph node. Reticular fibers (arrows) are present in the capsule (C), trabeculae (T), and substance of the organ, where they form a delicate internal framework. Silver stain. × 140.

FIGURE 2-24
Photomicrograph illustrating reticular fibers in the periphery of a lymph nodule and in the internodular area. Silver stain. × 344.

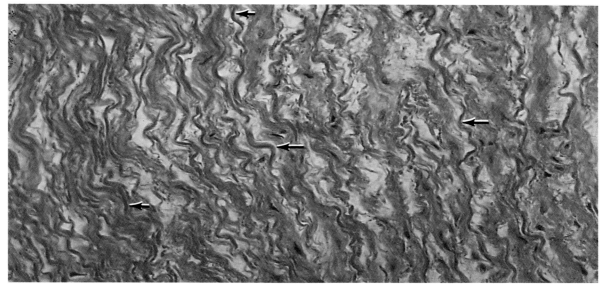

figure 2-22

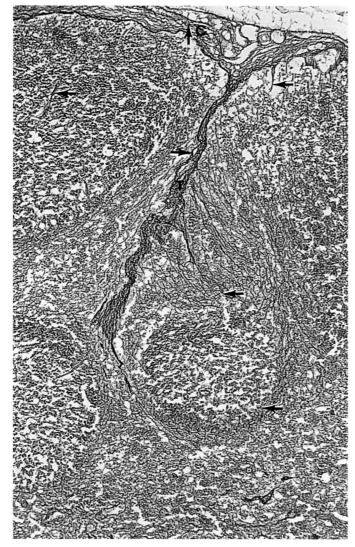

figure 2-23

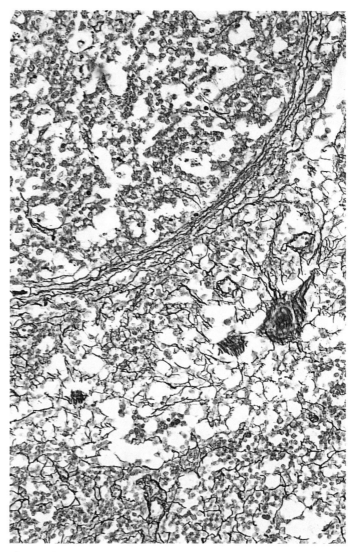

figure 2-24

3 Cartilage

FIGURE 3-1

Photomicrograph of hyaline cartilage from the trachea. Note the chondrocytes (c) in the avascular matrix (m). "Seemingly empty" lacunae (L) are a result of tissue processing. Isogenic groups (G) of chondrocytes occur within the matrix. The perichondrium (P) is dense irregular connective tissue. × 140.

FIGURE 3-2

Higher-power photomicrograph of hyaline cartilage demonstrating chondrocytes (C) and an empty lacuna (L) within the intercellular matrix (m). The more intensely stained material immediately around the chondrocytes is the territorial (capsular) matrix (T). The arrow is pointing to an isogenic clone. × 344.

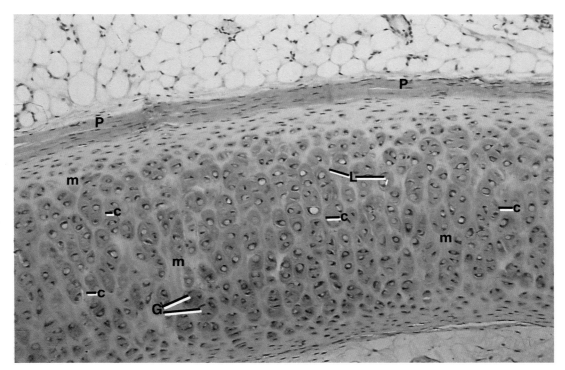

figure 3-1

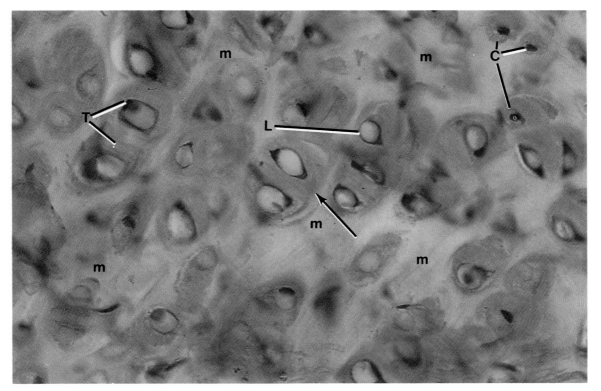

figure 3-2

FIGURE 3-3
Photomicrograph of elastic cartilage from the epiglottis showing elastic fibers enmeshing chondrocytes and obscuring the cartilage matrix (arrows). Elastic cartilage is avascular and has a perichondrium (P). Weigert's stain. × 140.

FIGURE 3-4
Photomicrograph of fibrocartilage from the symphysis pubis. The varying staining intensity of the matrix reflects varying densities of collagen (c) within the matrix. Isogenic groups of chondrocytes (arrows) are seen. Fibrocartilage is avascular and has no perichondrium. Masson's stain. × 140.

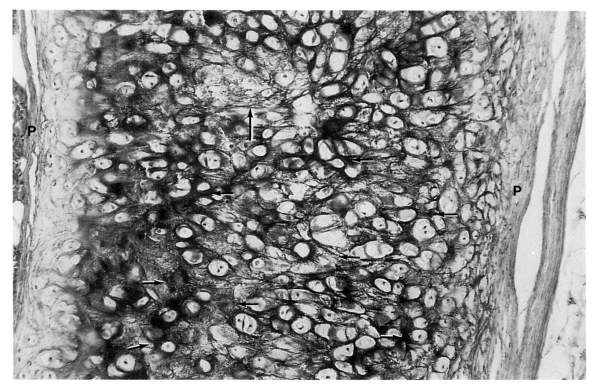

figure 3-3

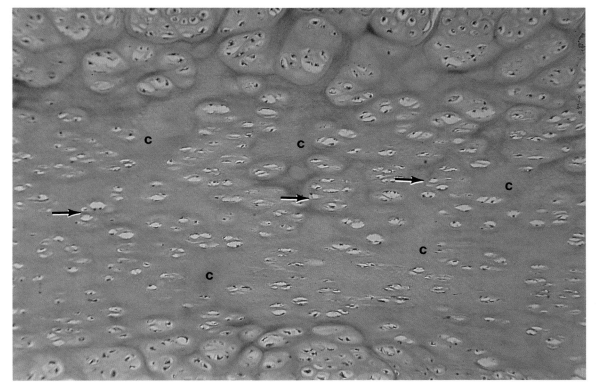

figure 3-4

FIGURE 3-5
Electron micrograph of a group of nine proteoglycan monomers extracted from hyaline cartilage. Shadow cast with platinum palladium. Rabbit; × 53,900.

FIGURE 3-6
Electron micrograph of a proteglycan aggregate extracted from hyaline cartilage. Note the hyaluronic acid backbone (H) and monomers (M). Shadow cast with platinum palladium. Rabbit; × 64,800.

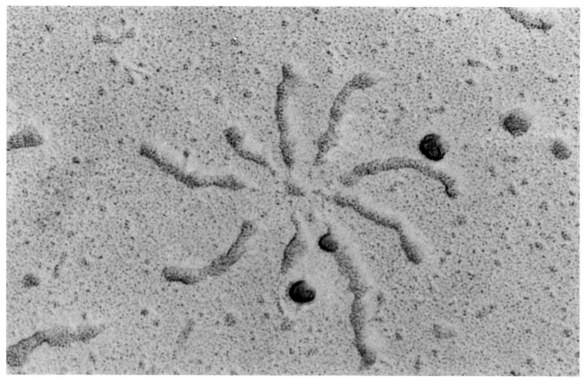

figure 3-5

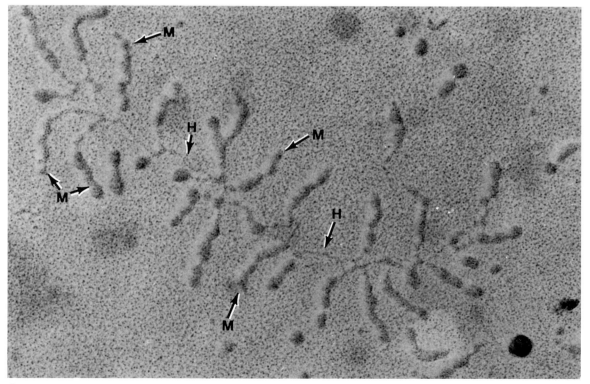

figure 3-6

4 Bone

FIGURE 4-1

Cross section of the diaphysis of a long bone (rabbit femur) showing the four organizational patterns of compact bone. Closest to the marrow cavity (M) are circularly arranged layers of bone, the inner circumferential lamellae (IC). The outer circumferential lamellae (OC) are circularly arranged layers of bone closest to skeletal muscle (S). Most typical and distinctive of compact bone are haversian systems (or osteons), lamellae of mineralized matrix with osteocytes (O) concentrically arranged around a vascular channel, the haversian (or central) canal (H). Between haversian systems are layers of bone called interstitial lamellae. Vascular channels which connect with haversian canals are Volkmann's canals (V). × 140.

FIGURE 4-2

Photomicrograph of cancellous bone of developing mouse jaw in which haversian systems are conspicuously absent. Simple squamous cells that line the surface of cancellous bone are inactive osteoprogenitors or bone-lining cells (BL) that give rise to cuboid-shaped osteoblasts (OB), which synthesize bone matrix. Cement lines (CL) demarcate regions where bone has been laid down appositionally. Note the osteocytes (O) and the numerous blood vessels (V) in the immediate vicinity of the trabeculae of bone. × 140.

FIGURE 4-3

Photomicrograph of cancellous bone of mouse jaw clearly illustrating the morphologic difference between inactive bone lining (endosteal, osteoprogenitor) cells (BL) and active osteoblasts (OB). The clear area between the osteoblasts and calcified bone represents unmineralized matrix or osteoid. CL, cement lines; O, osteocytes. × 344.

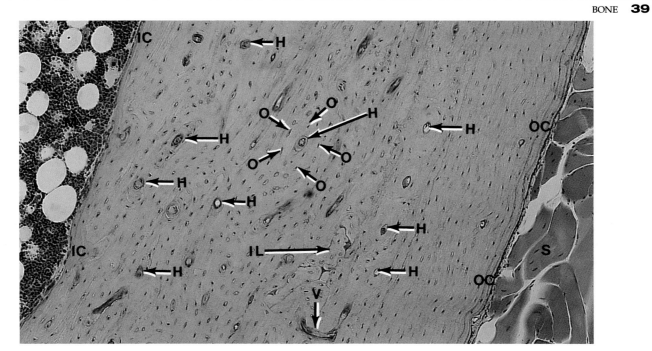

figure 4-1

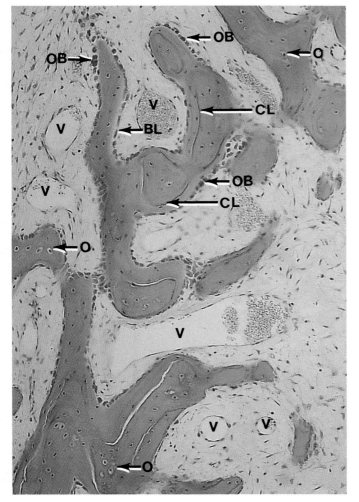

figure 4-2

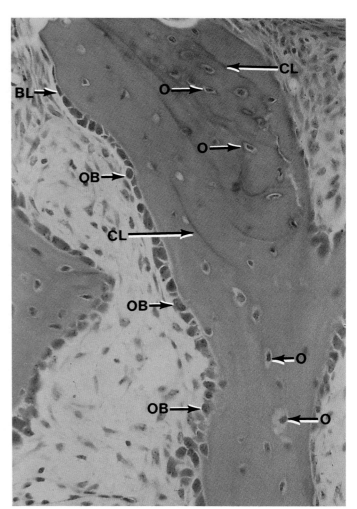

figure 4-3

FIGURE 4-4
Undecalcified ground section of compact bone depicting the structure of the osteon (haversian system). Note how the lamellae (L) of bone are concentrically arranged around the haversian (or central) canal (H). The thin dense lines represent canaliculi (C) that contain osteocyte (O) cell processes. Rabbit; × 560.

FIGURE 4-5
Cross section of decalcified compact bone with two complete haversian systems. Empty lacunae (L) are the result of slide preparation. Note the canaliculi (C) that radiate toward (or from) the haversian canal (H) but do not go beyond the cement line (CL), the outer limit of an osteon. IL, interstitial lamellae. Modified silver impregnation. Dog; × 560. (Courtesy of Mr. Ralph Alvarez.)

FIGURE 4-6
Photomicrograph illustrating the connection between a haversian canal (H) and Volkmann's canal (V). Modified silver impregnation. Dog; × 450. (Courtesy of Mr. Ralph Alvarez.)

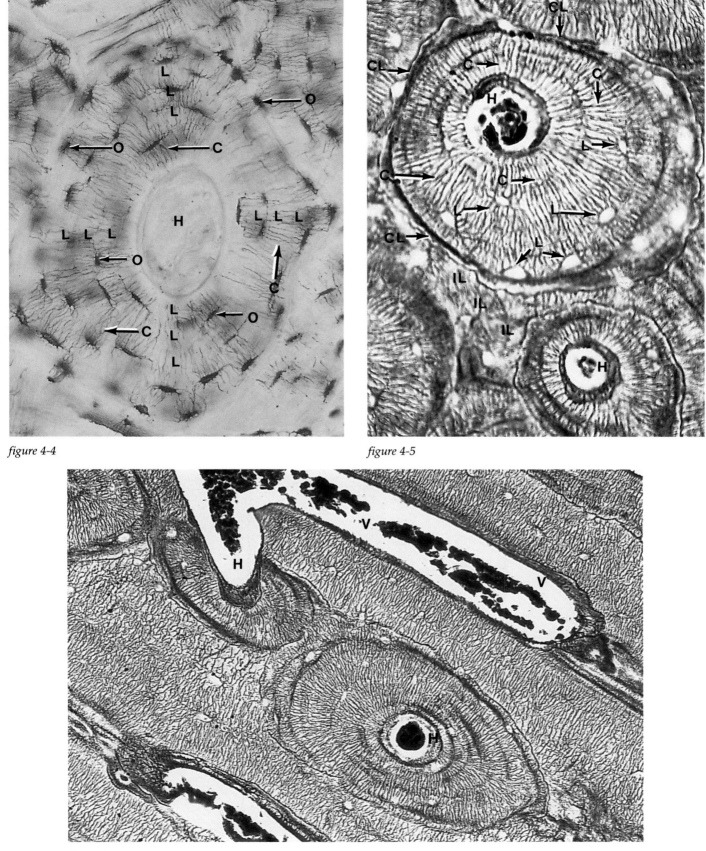

figure 4-4

figure 4-5

figure 4-6

FIGURE 4-7
Photomicrograph showing the bone-lining (endosteal) cells (BL) of compact bone and of Volkmann's canal. Also illustrated are the inner circumferential lamellae (IC), osteocytes (O), cement line (CL), and a mitotic figure (M) in bone marrow (BM). Rabbit; × 344.

FIGURE 4-8
Photomicrograph illustrating the bone-lining (osteoprogenitor) cells (BL) of the osteogenic layer of the periosteum (P). Note the cement lines (CL) of the outer circumferential lamellae (OC). O, osteocytes; S, skeletal muscle. Rabbit; × 344.

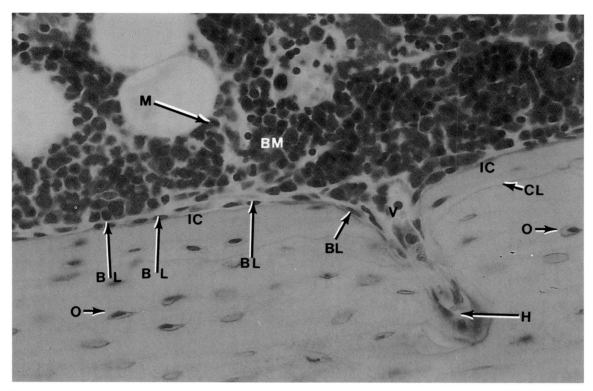

figure 4-7

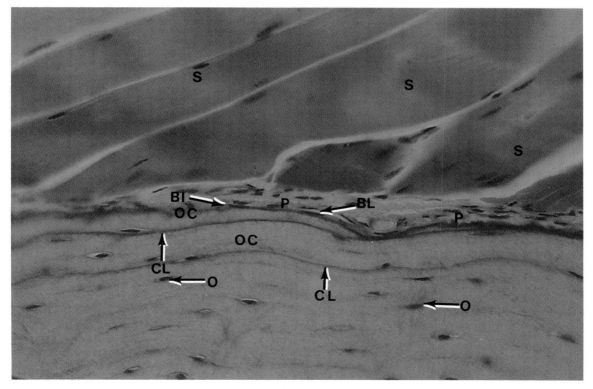

figure 4-8

FIGURE 4-9
Photomicrograph of an osteoclast (arrow) in Howship's lacunae (H). Note the ruffled border (RB) of the osteoclast. CT, connective tissue. Dog; × 450. Modified silver stain counterstained with fast green–metanil yellow mixture. (Courtesy of Mr. Ralph Alvarez.)

FIGURE 4-10
Photomicrograph of an osteoclast (arrow). Note the part of the cell's ruffled border (RB) which is still attached to the surface of bone. H, Howship's lacunae. Modified silver stain counterstained with fast green–metanil yellow mixture. Dog; × 560. (Courtesy of Mr. Ralph Alvarez.)

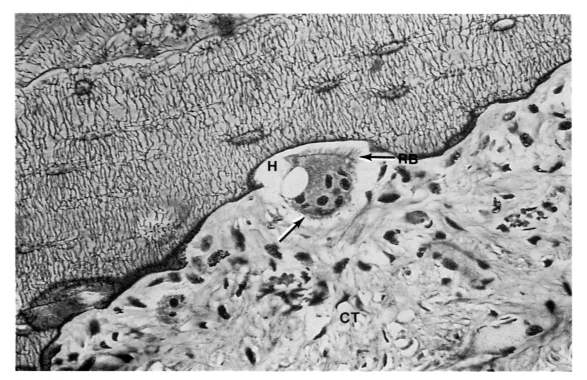

figure 4-9

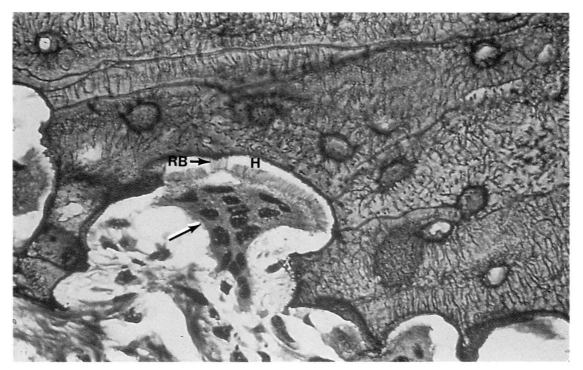

figure 4-10

5 Bone Formation

FIGURE 5-1

Low-power photomicrograph of long-bone formation by the process of endochondral ossification. Apparent are the epiphyseal growth plate (GP), trabeculae of mineralized tissue (T), perichondrium (P) of epiphyseal hyaline cartilage (E), periosteum of diaphyseal bone (PE), and developing synovial capsule (S). Note the blood vessels (V) in the otherwise avascular hyaline cartilage of the epiphysis (E) presaging the development of secondary centers of ossification. M, medullary (marrow) cavity. × 14.

FIGURE 5-2

Endochondral ossification in developing mouse phalange. Note the difference in morphology of the two epiphyseal growth plates (GP). Also apparent are resting (R), proliferating (P), hypertrophic (H), and calcified cartilage (C) zones. M, medullary (marrow) cavity. × 56.

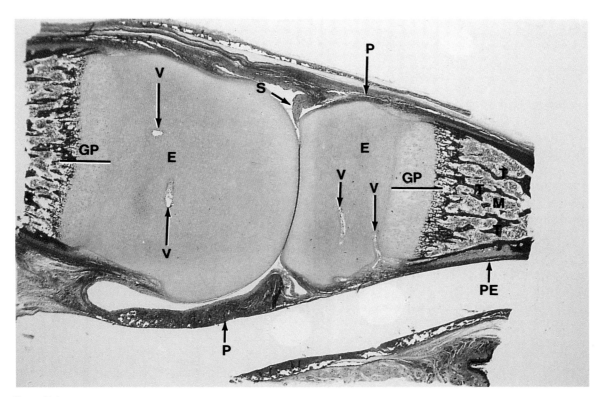

figure 5-1

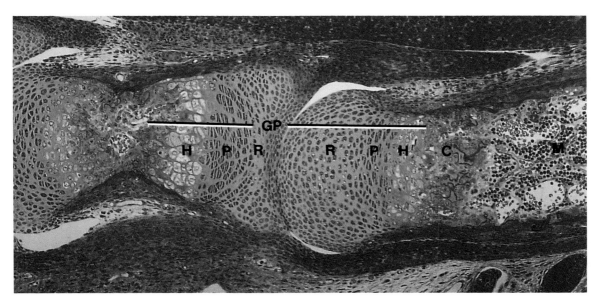

figure 5-2

FIGURE 5-3

Low-power photomicrograph illustrating a more advanced stage of endochondral bone formation than that shown in Figure 5-2. Note the epiphysial growth plate (GP) with resting (R), proliferating (P), and hypertrophic (H) zones, and the calcified cell (C) zone, which stains purple in this preparation. Note also the mineralized tissue in the medullary (marrow) cavity (M), which is an admixture of bone (B) and calcified cartilage (C). Rabbit; × 56.

FIGURE 5-4

Higher-power view of the hypertrophic (H) cell zone and zone of calcified cartilage (C) of the epiphyseal growth plate seen in Figure 5-3. Note the seams of calcified cartilage in the bone (B) of the medullary (marrow) cavity (M). Rabbit; × 140.

FIGURE 5-5

Photomicrograph clearly illustrating the core of calcified cartilage (C) upon which bone (B) has been laid down. M, medullary (marrow) cavity. Rabbit; × 140.

FIGURE 5-6

Photomicrograph of diaphyseal bone (B) with a well-developed periosteum (P), the inner cells of which are bone-lining (osteoprogenitor) cells (BL). C, calcified cartilage; M, medullary (marrow) cavity. Rabbit; × 140.

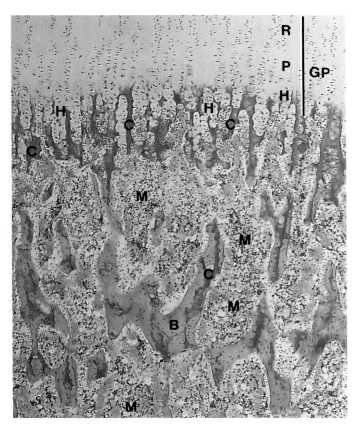

figure 5-3

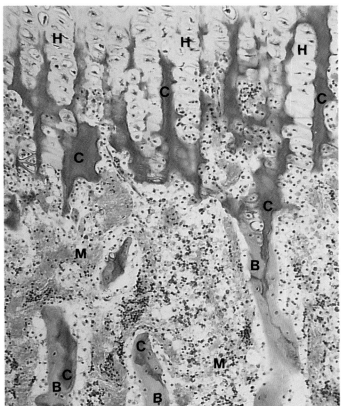

figure 5-4

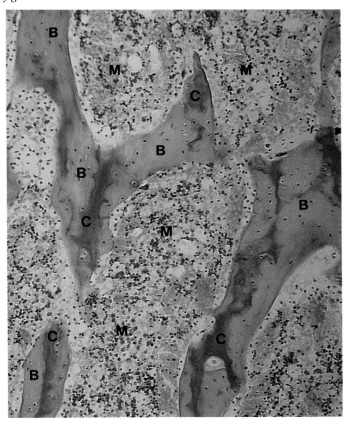

figure 5-5

figure 5-6

Figures 5-7 through 5-9: Intramembranous bone formation. Note particularly the absence of any calcified cartilage in areas of forming bone.

FIGURE 5-7

Low-power photomicrograph illustrating cancellous bone (B) that has formed in an area of mesenchymal tissue (M). Note the region of more condensed mesenchyme (CM) and the numerous osteoblasts (O) that line the trabeculae of bone (BL). V, blood vessels. Pig jaw; × 56.

FIGURE 5-8

Photomicrograph illustrating numerous trabeculae of cancellous bone (B) initially produced by intramembranous formation. Both bone-lining (osteoprogenitor) cells (BL) and osteoblasts (O) are present on the surface of the trabeculae of cancellous bone. Note the extensive vascularity (V) in close proximity to the developing bone. M, mesenchyme. Pig jaw; × 140.

FIGURE 5-9

Photomicrograph of intramembranous bone formation depicting the development of a periosteum (P) and suggesting the conversion of cancellous bone (B) to compact bone by the entrapment of blood vessels (V) within the bone by osteoblastic (O) activity. M, mesenchyme. Pig jaw; × 140.

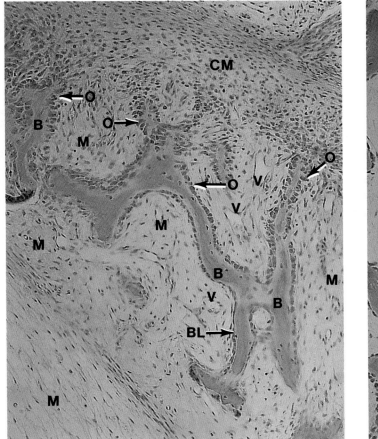

figure 5-7

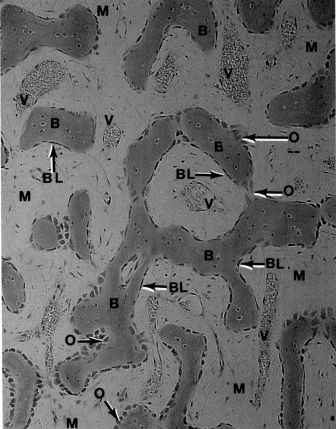

figure 5-8

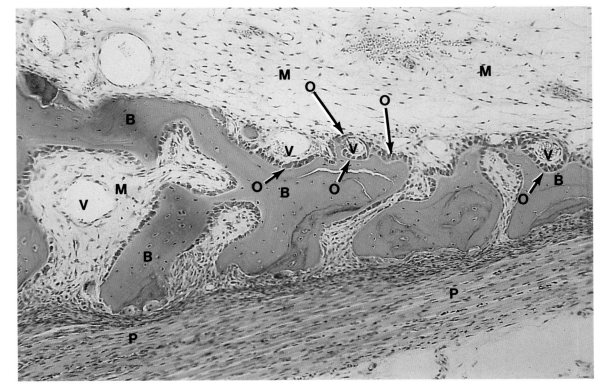

figure 5-9

FIGURE 6-1

Photomicrograph illustrating the relationship between the spinal cord and nerve fibers of the dorsal (F) and ventral (V) roots. The spinal cord is divided into white matter (W), dorsal gray (DG), and ventral gray (VG) matter. Note the central canal (C) of the spinal cord, the dorsal root ganglion (D), and intervertebral disc (ID). Luxol blue stain. Immature rabbit; × 11.

FIGURE 6-2

Photomicrograph depicting the molecular (M) and granular (G) layers of the gray matter of the cerebellum. Between the molecular and granular layers is the thin Purkinje cell layer (P) just discernible in this micrograph. W, white matter of the cerebellum. Luxol blue stain. Rabbit; × 11.

FIGURE 6-3

Photomicrograph of a cross section of gyri of the cerebral cortex illustrating the region encompassing the six cell layers of the cerebral cortex (C) and underlying white matter (W). Note the vasculature (V), corpus callosum (CC), and fornix (F). Gallocyanin stain. Rhesus monkey; × 11.

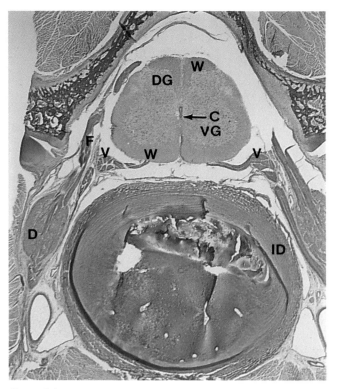

figure 6-1

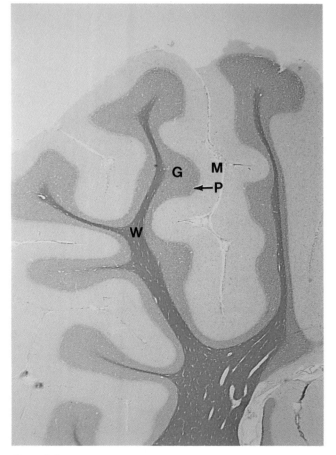

figure 6-2

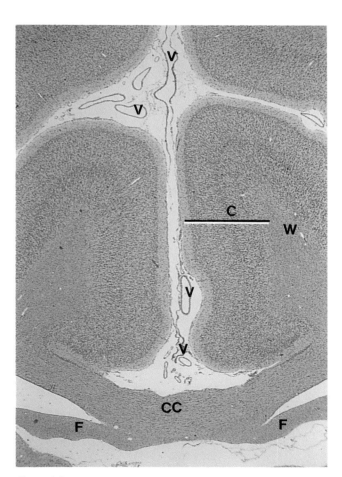

figure 6-3

FIGURE 6-4
Photomicrograph of a motor neuron showing the nucleolus (NU), Nissl bodies (NB), axon hillock (AH), axon (A), dendrites (D), and blood vessel (V). × 869.

FIGURE 6-5
Photomicrograph of a section of ventral gray matter depicting motor neurons and nerve fibers (F). N, nucleus of motor neuron; (NU), nucleolus; L, lipofuscin pigment. The clear space between the neurons and fibers is an artifact of slide preparation. Luxol blue stain. × 344.

FIGURE 6-6
Photomicrograph of a cross section of ventral gray matter stained with silver. N, nucleus of motor neuron; NU, nucleolus; F, nerve fibers; L, lipofuscin pigment. The space between the neurons and nerve fibers is an artifact of slide preparation. Silver stain. × 344.

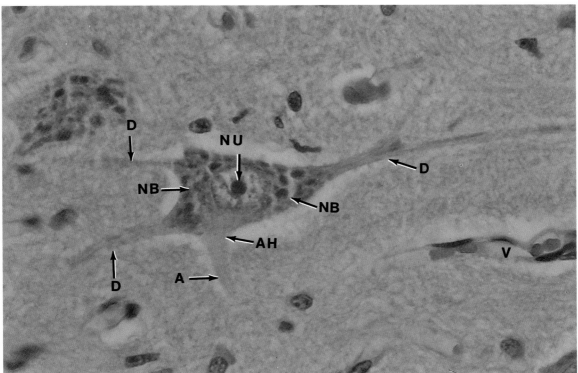

figure 6-4

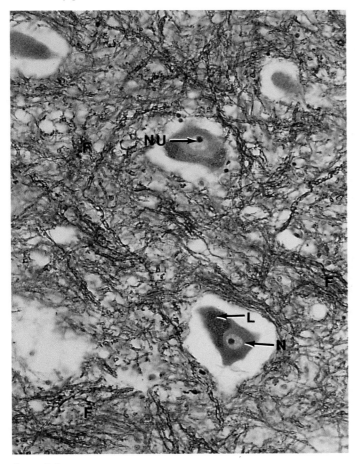

figure 6-5

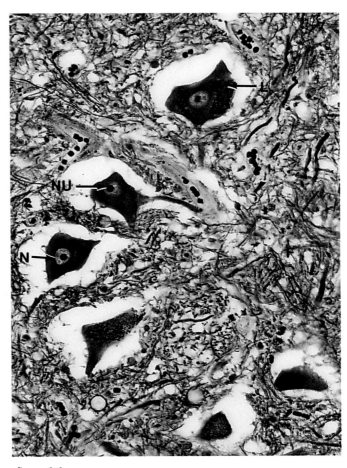

figure 6-6

FIGURE 6-7
Photomicrograph illustrating the morphologic difference between neuronal cells (N) and support (neuroglial) cells (G) of the central nervous system. Gallocyanin stain. Rhesus monkey; × 344.

FIGURE 6-8
Photomicrograph of a Purkinje cell from the cerebellum. S, soma (cell body); P, cell processes. Silver stain. × 560.

FIGURE 6-9
Photomicrograph of protoplasmic astrocytes from the gray matter of the spinal cord. S, soma (cell body); P, cell processes. Gold chloride stain. × 560.

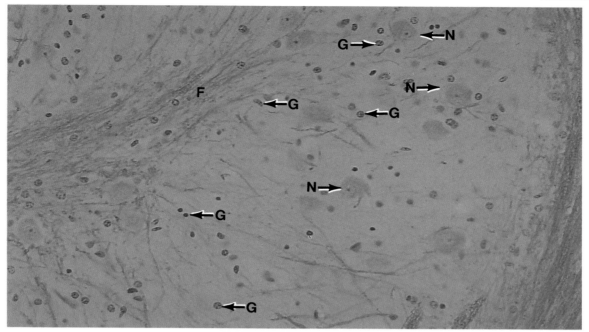

figure 6-7

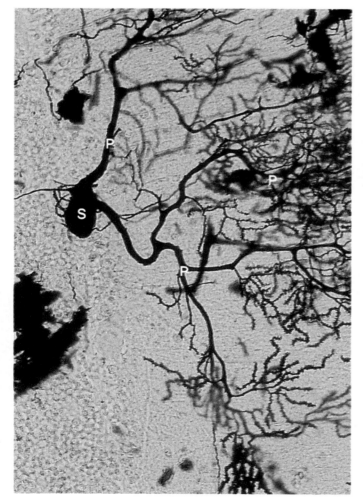

figure 6-8

figure 6-9

FIGURE 6-10
Photomicrograph of a dorsal root (sensory) ganglion (G) in the peripheral nervous system. Note the nerve fibers (F) coursing through the ganglion and the connective tissue capsule (C) surrounding the ganglion. Luxol blue stain. Immature rabbit; × 56.

FIGURE 6-11
Photomicrograph of dorsal root (sensory) ganglion cells. Apparent are the nucleus (N) and nucleolus (NU) of the ganglion cells, satellite cells (S), and lipofuscin (L). × 560.

FIGURE 6-12
Photomicrograph of sympathetic ganglion cells in the peripheral nervous system showing the nucleus (N) of a ganglion cell, satellite cells (S), and the capsule (C) of the ganglion. The space between a part of the nerve fascicle (N) and its perineurium (P) is an artifact of slide preparation. L, lipofuscin. × 344.

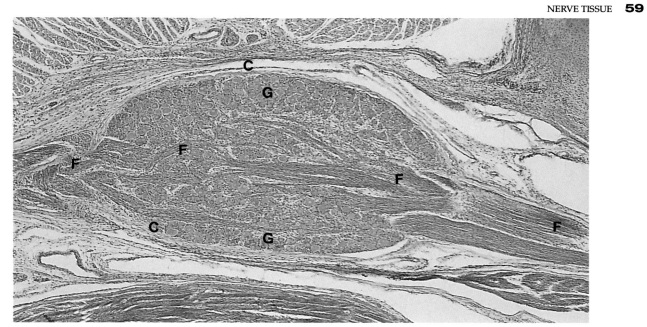

figure 6-10

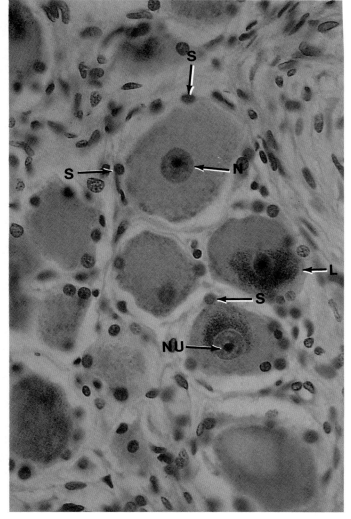

figure 6-11

figure 6-12

FIGURE 6-13
Electron micrograph of two sensory ganglion nerve cells. N, nucleus; NU, nucleolus; M, mitochondria; L, lysosomes. Rat; × 6375. (Reproduced from *Journal of Cell Biology,* 1967, vol. 32, pp. 439–466, by copyright permission of the Rockefeller University Press. Courtesy of Dr. Mary Bartlett Bunge et al.)

FIGURE 6-14
Electron micrograph illustrating the satellite cell covering of a dorsal root ganglion cell. S, satellite cell covering cytoplasm; N, nucleus of ganglion cell; G, Golgi; L, lysosomes. Rat; × 6375. (Reproduced from *Journal of Cell Biology,* 1967, vol. 32, pp. 439–466, by copyright permission of the Rockefeller University Press. Courtesy of Dr. Mary Bartlett Bunge et al.)

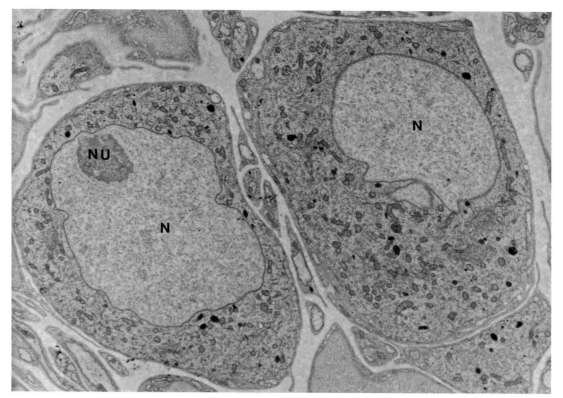

figure 6-13

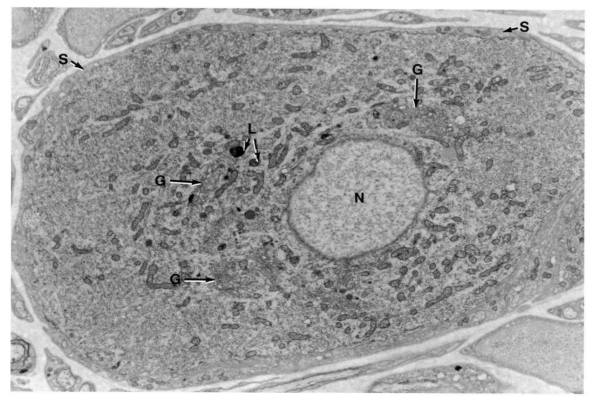

figure 6-14

FIGURE 6-15
Photomicrograph of a peripheral nerve bundle depicting its outer connective tissue covering the epineurium (E) and perineurium (P) of nerve fascicles (N). Note the artery (A) and vein (V). Pig; × 140.

FIGURE 6-16
Photomicrograph of a cross section of a nerve bundle illustrating the endoneurium of nerve fibers (E). A, axon; M, myelin sheath. Silver stain. × 344.

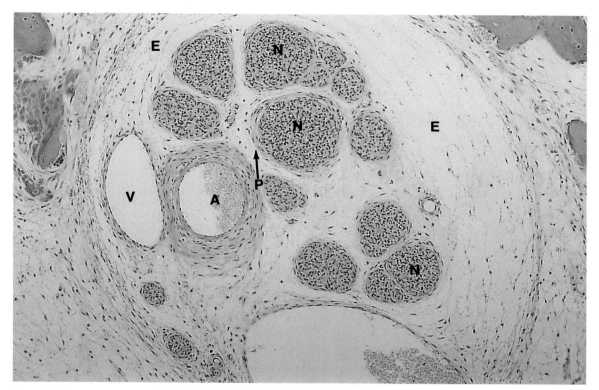

figure 6-15

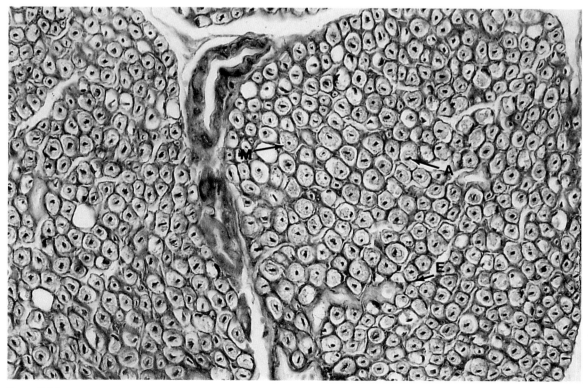

figure 6-16

FIGURE 6-17
Photomicrograph of the perineurium (P) encompassing a small nerve fascicle (N) separating it from two other fascicles (N). × 344.

FIGURE 6-18
Photomicrograph of a solitary nerve fascicle surrounded by its perineurium (P). Note the endoneurium (E) surrounding a nerve fiber. × 344.

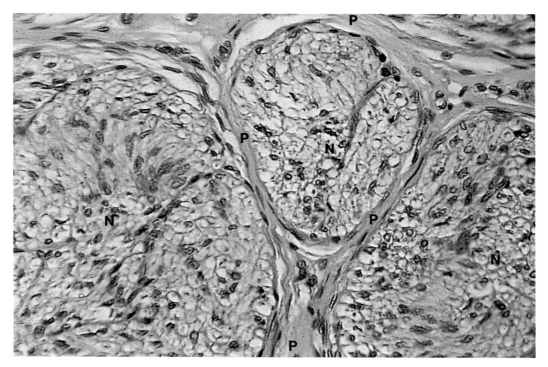

figure 6-17

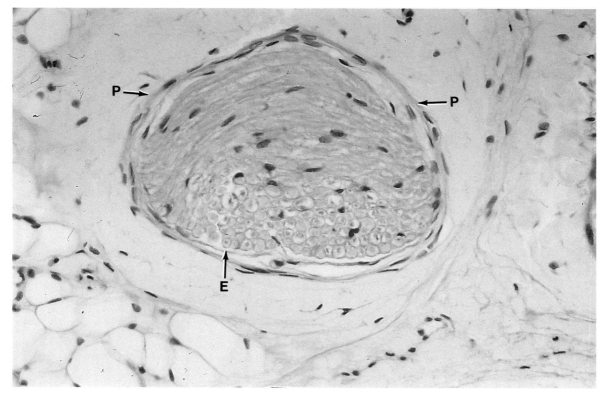

figure 6-18

FIGURE 6-19
Photomicrograph of a longitudinally sectioned nerve fascicle. Note the thin fusiform profiles of fibroblasts (F) of the endoneurium and plumper profiles of Schwann cells (S). P, perineurium. × 344.

FIGURE 6-20
Photomicrograph of a single myelinated nerve fiber illustrating the node of Ranvier (N). Note the interruption in the myelin sheath (M) where the axon (A) crosses the node. E, endoneurium. Osmium stain. × 869.

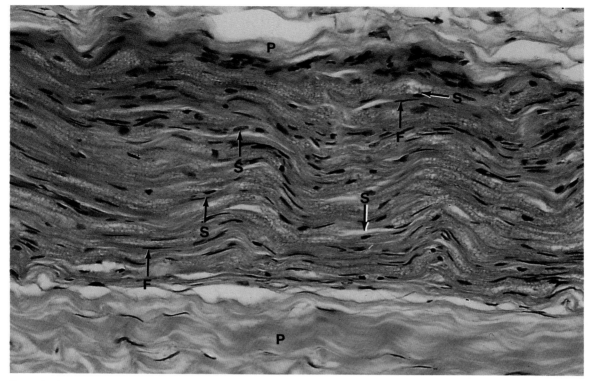

figure 6-19

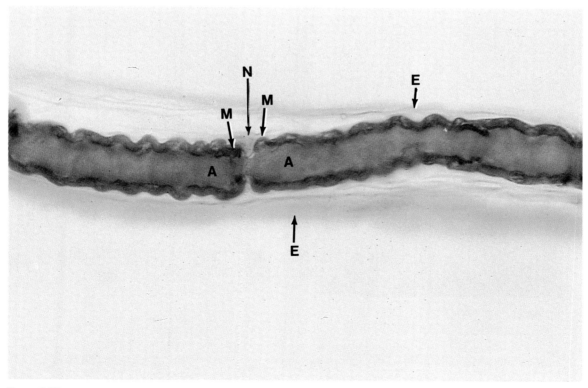

figure 6-20

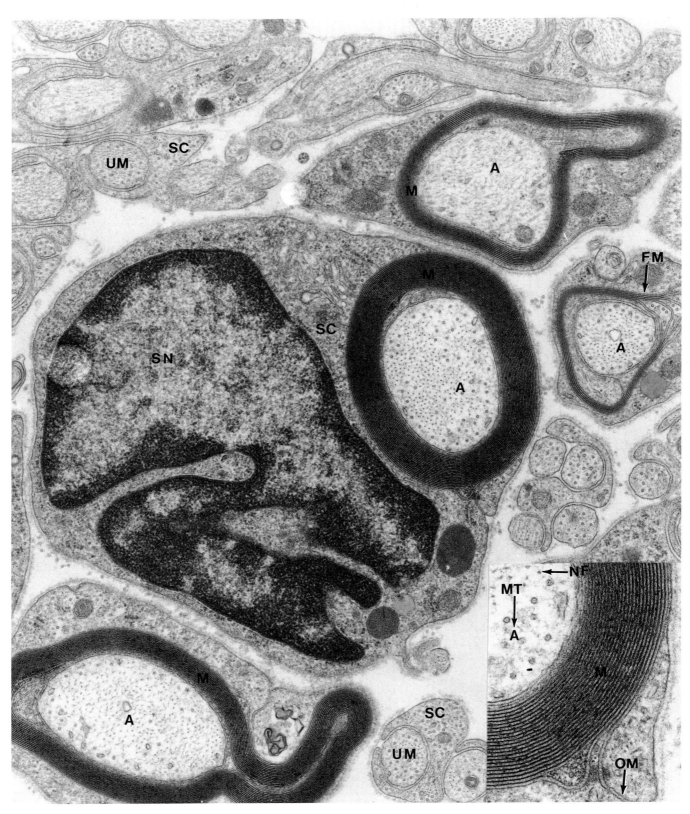

FIGURE 6-21

Electron micrograph illustrating myelinated and unmyelinated peripheral nerve fibers. SN, Schwann cell nucleus; SC, Schwann cell cytoplasm; M, myelin sheath; FM, forming myelin sheath; UM, unmyelinated axon. Rat; × 28,420. **Inset:** Electron micrograph of part of a myelinated axon depicting the outer mesaxon (OM), myelin sheath (M), neurofilaments (NF), and microtubules (MT) cut in cross section. Rat; × 69,580. (Courtesy of Dr. Mary Bartlett Bunge.)

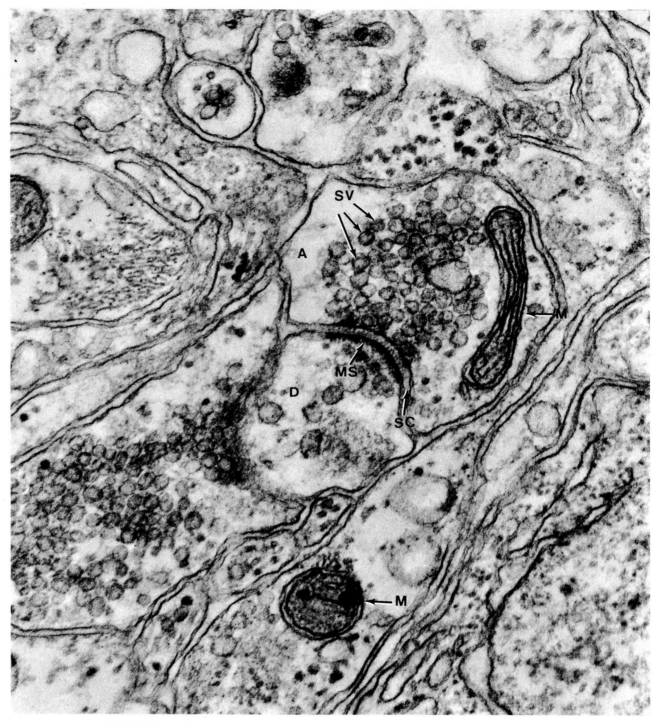

FIGURE 6-22

Electron micrograph of an axodendritic synapse showing the axon (A), dendrite (D), synaptic vesicles (SV), membrane specialization (MS), synaptic cleft (SC), and mitochondria (M). Rat; × 99,000. (Reproduced from *Journal of Cell Biology,* 1965, vol. 24, pp. 163–191, by copyright permission of the Rockefeller University Press. Courtesy of Dr. Richard Bunge, Dr. Mary Bartlett Bunge, and Dr. Edith R. Peterson.)

FIGURE 7-1
Photomicrograph illustrating the major morphologic features of skeletal muscle cut in cross and longitudinal section. In the longitudinally cut fiber (L), note the cross striations (S) and the peripheral location of multinuclei (N). Nuclei (N) are also peripherally located in cross sectioned fibers (X). Also shown are an arteriole (A) and fibroblast nuclei (F) in the surrounding connective tissue (C). G, serous glands. × 344.

FIGURE 7-2
Photomicrograph of thin longitudinally sectioned skeletal muscle illustrating alternating dark (A) and light (I) transverse striations, which represent respectively the A and I bands of skeletal muscle. Note the peripheral location of nuclei (N) of the muscle fibers and the nuclei of fibroblasts (F) of the endomysium. × 560.

FIGURE 7-3
Photomicrograph of portions of two skeletal muscle fascicles cut in cross section. Separating the fascicles is the connective tissue of the perimysium (P). As a consequence of shrinkage of muscle cells during slide preparation, the endomysium (E), the connective tissue covering of individual muscle fibers, can be visualized. Note the cross-sectioned fibers, some of which display multiple nuclei peripherally located (X). × 140.

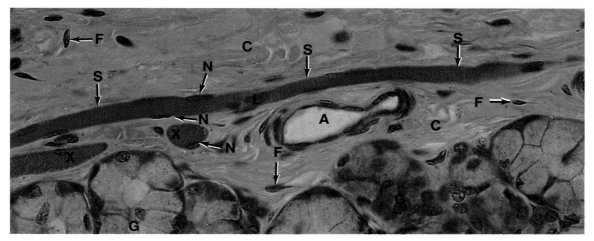

figure 7-1

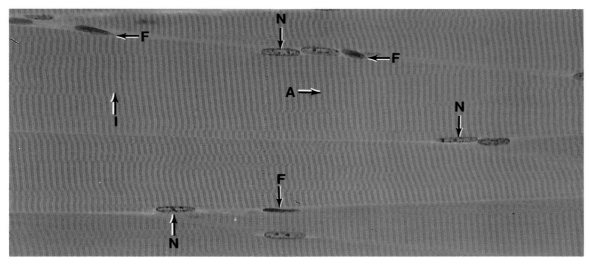

figure 7-2

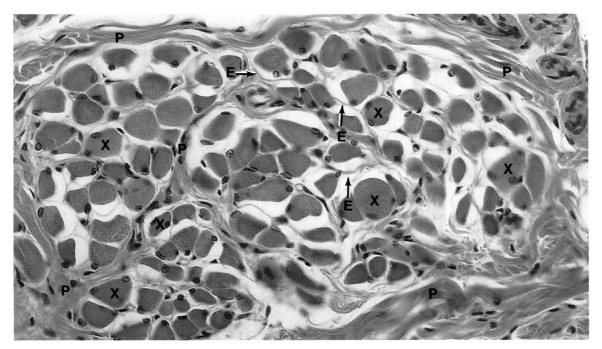

figure 7-3

FIGURE 7-4

Electron micrograph of a skeletal muscle fiber illustrating the alignment of myofibrils that results in the morphology of skeletal muscle observed in light microscopy. The contractile unit of the fiber, the sarcomere, is delineated by two Z lines (Z), which bisect the I band (I). Within the sarcomere is an electron-dense A band (A) bisected by an electron-translucent H band (H). Note the triads (arrows) and mitochondria (M). Rat; × 24,280. (Courtesy of Dr. Mikel Snow.)

FIGURE 7-5

Electron micrograph of a skeletal muscle satellite cell cut in cross section. Note that the satellite cell (S) lies completely within the external lamina (EL) of the muscle fiber (MF) at the bottom of the micrograph. N, nucleus of muscle fiber; M, mitochondria; CP, cell process of capillary endothelial cell; E, erythrocyte. Rat; × 25,600. (Courtesy of Dr. Mikel Snow.)

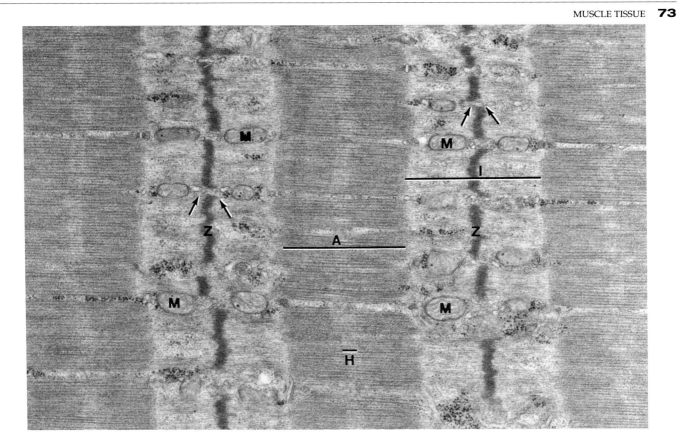

figure 7-4

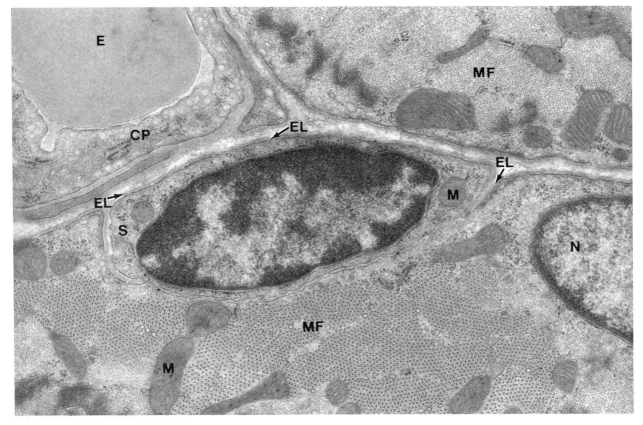

figure 7-5

FIGURE 7-6

Photomicrograph depicting the termination of a motor neuron in a motor end plate (MEP) of a skeletal muscle fiber (S). NF, nerve fibers. Silver impregnation counterstained with metanil yellow. Rat; × 430. (Courtesy of Mr. Ralph Alvarez.)

FIGURE 7-7

Electron micrograph of a muscle spindle. Illustrated are four intrafusial muscle fibers (MF) surrounded by a laminated connective tissue capsule (C). SC, satellite cells of muscle fibers; MA, myelinated axon. × 3600. (Courtesy of Dr. Mikel Snow.)

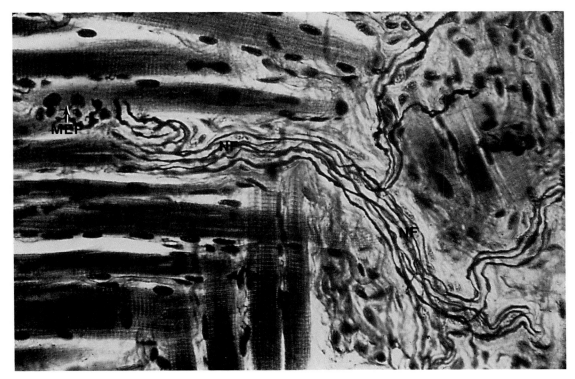

figure 7-6

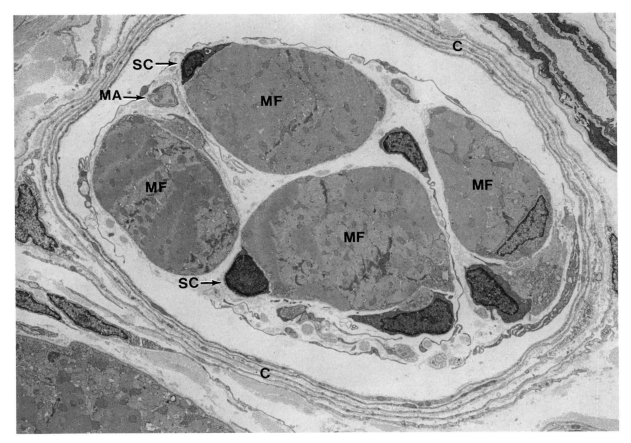

figure 7-7

FIGURE 7-8
Photomicrograph of cardiac muscle illustrating centrally located nuclei (N) in longitudinally cut striated fibers (S). Note the reticular fibers (R) that surround individual cardiac muscle fibers. C, collagen. Plastic section. Cat; × 430. Variation of Ortega's reticular stain. (Courtesy of Mr. Ralph Alvarez.)

FIGURE 7-9
Low-power electron micrograph of cardiac muscle illustrating typical features of striated muscle. The Z line (Z) bisects the I band (I) and represents the boundaries of a sarcomere. The A band (A) is bisected by the H band (H). Note the intercalated disc (arrow), a distinguishing morphologic feature of cardiac muscle. M, mitochondria; D, diads of the tubular system. Rat; × 5500. (Courtesy of Mr. Jean-Pierre Brunschwig.)

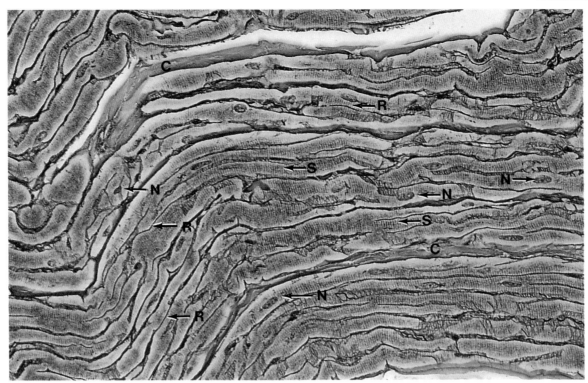

figure 7-8

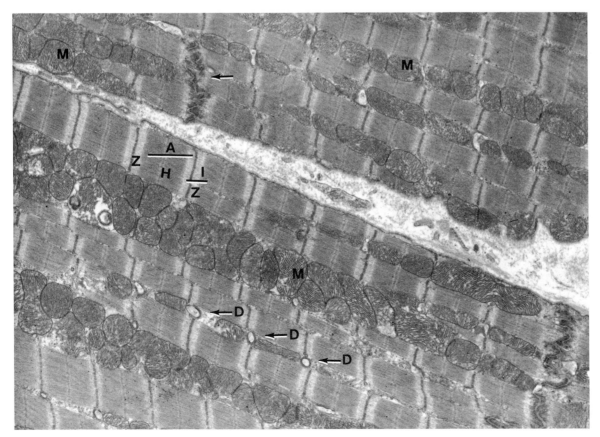

figure 7-9

FIGURE 7-10
Photomicrograph depicting intercalated discs (I), centrally located nuclei (N), and striations (S) of cardiac muscle. × 344.

FIGURE 7-11
Electron micrograph illustrating an intercalated disc (arrows). Note the macula adherens (desmosome) (D) and fascia adherens (F). M, mitochondria. Rat; × 31,730. (Courtesy of Ms. Susan Decker.)

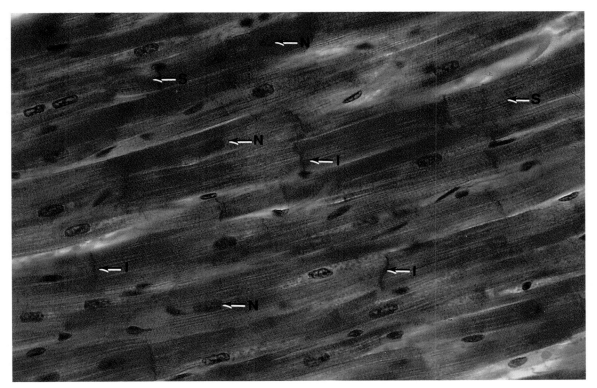

figure 7-10

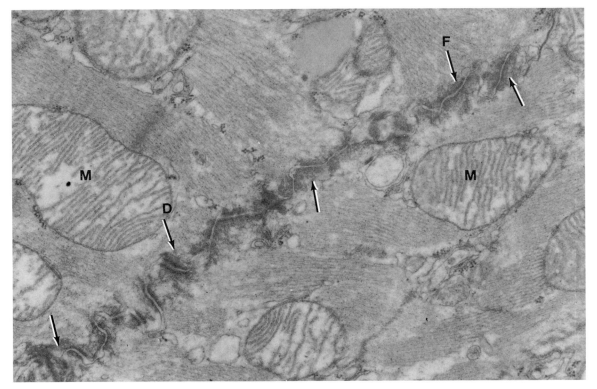

figure 7-11

FIGURE 7-12
Photomicrograph illustrating the nuclei (arrows) of the inner circular (IC) and outer longitudinal (OL) layers of smooth muscle of the small intestine when cut in cross section. C, connective tissue. × 140.

FIGURE 7-13
Photomicrograph depicting the nuclei of smooth muscle cells (arrows) cut in longitudinal section in the tunica media of a small artery. C, connective tissue of the adventitial coat of the vessel. × 140.

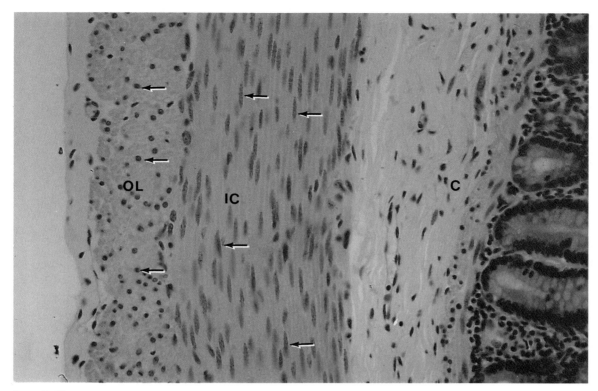

figure 7-12

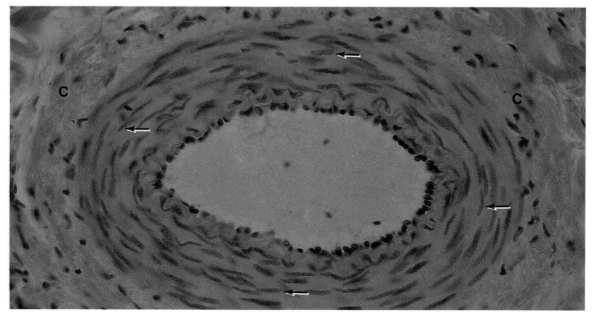

figure 7-13

8 Formed Elements of Blood

FIGURE 8-1

Neutrophil (N), monocyte (M), and lymphocyte (L). Note the segmented nucleus of the neutrophil, the horseshoe-shaped nucleus of the monocyte, and the oval nucleus of the lymphocyte. The cytoplasm of the neutrophil appears lightly granular, whereas that of the monocyte and lymphocyte appears agranular; the latter stains more basophilic. The anucleate cells in the background are erythrocytes with a pale-staining central region due to their biconcave disc shape. Wright's stain. × 896.

FIGURE 8-2

Neutrophil (N) and eosinophil (E). Note the coarse reddish-orange-stained cytoplasmic granules that characterize eosinophils and the lightly stained fine granules of the neutrophil. Nuclei of eosinophils are typically bilobed. Nuclei of neutrophils may contain as many as five lobes. Wright's stain. × 1376.

FIGURE 8-3

Neutrophil (N) and lymphocyte (L). Note the highly lobulated nucleus of the neutrophil and faintly stained granules in the cytoplasm. A Barr body (accessory chromosome) is evident (arrow) in this neutrophil from a female. The nucleus of the lymphocyte is nonlobulated, and the cytoplasm of the cell is not stained as basophilic as the lymphocyte shown in Figure 8-5. Wright's stain. × 1376.

FIGURE 8-4

A typical eosinophil (E) showing coarse orange-reddish cytoplasmic granules and a bilobed nucleus. Wright's stain. × 1376.

FIGURE 8-5

A lymphocyte (L) displaying lightly basophilic cytoplasm and an oval nucleus, which typifies the cell. Wright's stain. × 1376.

FIGURE 8-6

A monocyte (M) displaying a large indented nucleus and pale-staining cytoplasm with no visible granulation. Wright's stain. × 1376.

FIGURE 8-7

A basophil (B), the most distinctive cell in the circulation, showing coarse basophilic cytoplasmic granules that usually obscure the nucleus. Wright's stain. × 1376.

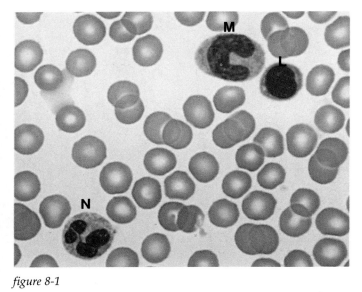

figure 8-1

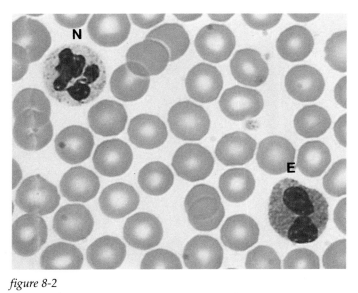

figure 8-2

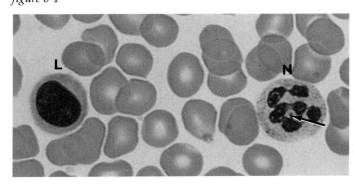

figure 8-3

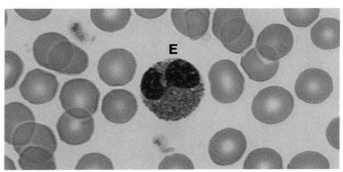

figure 8-4

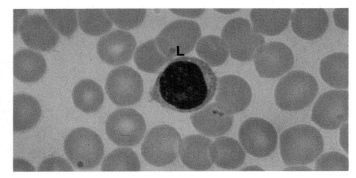

figure 8-5

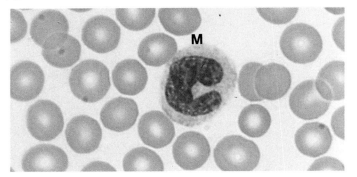

figure 8-6

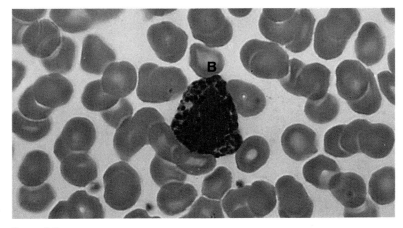

figure 8-7

FIGURE 8-8
Photomicrograph of reticulocytes (arrows). The densely staining material within the cell is ribosomal RNA stained by brilliant cresyl blue. × 1376.

FIGURE 8-9
Photomicrograph of platelets (arrows) and a clump of platelets (paired arrows). Wright's stain. × 1376.

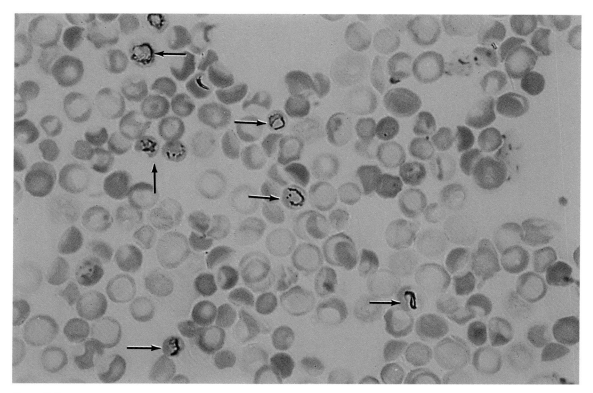

figure 8-8

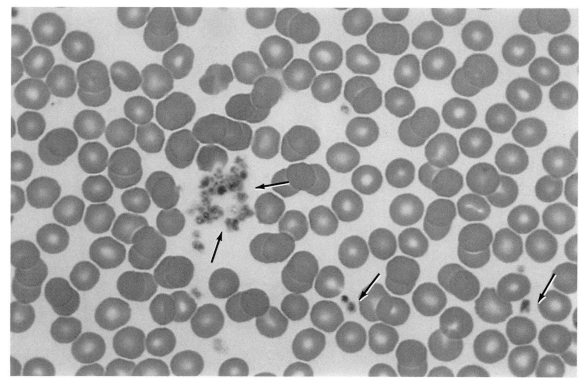

figure 8-9

FIGURE 8-10
Electron micrograph of a platelet (P) in bone marrow. Note the concentration of granules in the region called the granulomere (arrows) and the clearer peripheral area called the hyalomere of the platelet (H). Mouse marrow; × 12,936.

FIGURE 8-11
Electron micrograph of a platelet illustrating the granules of the granulomere (arrows) and the granule-free peripheral region of the hyalomere (H). Mouse blood; × 14,850.

FIGURE 8-12
Electron micrograph illustrating platelet agglutination in the lumen of a marrow sinusoid. Note the clumped and degranulated platelets (arrows) in association with collagen (C). EP, cell process of an endothelial cell of the marrow sinusoid. Mouse marrow; × 7546.

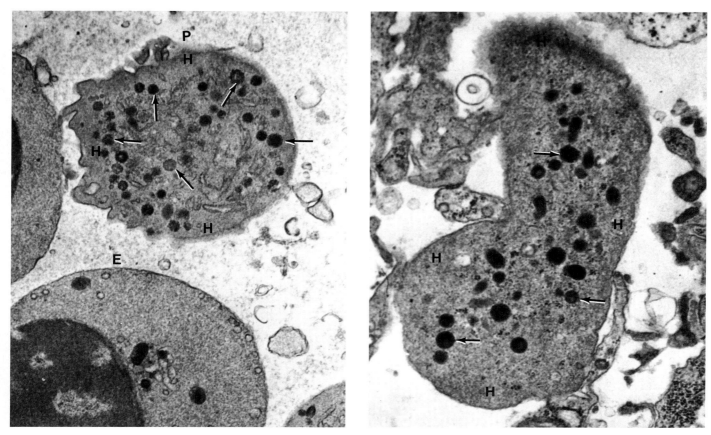

figure 8-10

figure 8-11

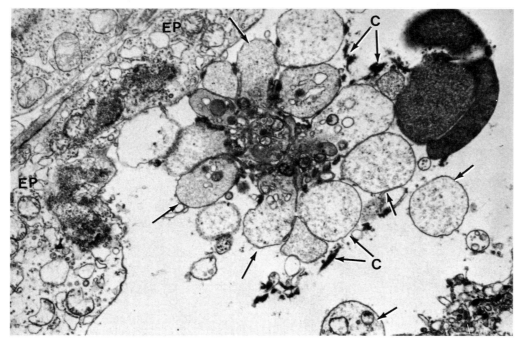

figure 8-12

GRANULOPOIESIS

The major morphologic changes that are important in recognizing the different stages in the maturation sequence of developing granulocytes involve

1. Development of specific cytoplasmic granules, which allows for recognition of cells in the eosinophilic, basophilic, or neutrophilic cell series.
2. Changes in nuclear shape, which coupled with the above allow for the placement of a cell in a specific maturational stage within the eosinophilic, basophilic, or neutrophilic cell series.

The first recognizable and most immature cell in the granulocytic series is the **myeloblast.** The myeloblast (14–16 μm) has an oval nucleus with finely dispersed chromatin (nucleoli may or may not be evident) and a thin rim of **slightly basophilic cytoplasm that is devoid of granules.**

The myeloblast, which gives rise to the **promyelocyte,** the largest cell (17–26 μm) in the series, has a large oval nucleus with finely dispersed chromatin and multiple nucleoli. The most prominent feature of the **promyelocyte** is the **abundant azurophilic granules** in its **cytoplasm.**

The promyelocyte gives rise to three types of **myelocytes,** each having **specific cytoplasmic granules of lilac (neutrophilic), orange to red (eosinophilic), or deep blue (basophilic) color,** which represent respectively **neutrophilic, eosinophilic, and basophilic myelocytes.** In early neutrophilic myelocytes, azurophilic granules appear to predominate in the cytoplasm as a result of the paucity and faint staining of neutrophilic granules. In more mature neutrophilic myelocytes, there are fewer azurophilic granules and the fine granular nature and lilac-staining qualities of neutrophilic granules are more apparent. The distinctive orange to red color of granules in the eosinophilic myelocyte and the deep blue coloration of granules in the basophilic myelocyte make it easy to distinguish these cells from each other and from neutrophilic myelocytes. Additional features of myelocytes are their size (10–18 μm), a moderately clumped **round** to **oval nucleus** with observable nucleoli, and a nuclear-to-cytoplasmic ratio favoring the cytoplasm, particularly in the more mature cells in this stage of development.

Each of the three types of myelocytes gives rise to cells called **metamyelocytes.** Metamyelocytes are characterized by a distinctive **change** in **nuclear morphology** from round or slightly oval to an **indented or kidney shape.** In addition, the nucleus of metamyelocytes is more clumped, and the nuclear to cytoplasmic ratio definitely favors the cytoplasm. Metamyelocytes are approximately the same size (10–15 μm) as or slightly smaller than myelocytes.

Metamyelocytes do not undergo mitosis but differentiate into cells called **band granulocytes.** These cells are characterized by **marked condensation** of the **nucleus,** which, as the name implies, assumes a **band shape.** The cell size (10–15 μm) is the same as that of the metamyelocyte.

Further maturation of band cells gives rise to the three types of granulocytes found in circulating blood, which are characterized by nuclei, segmented into lobes connected by thin strands of chromatin as well as cytoplasmic granules that are specific for the neutrophilic, eosinophilic, or basophilic cell series.

Examples of different stages in the development of cells in the neutrophilic and eosinophilic granulocyte cell series are illustrated in Figures 9-1–9-5.

ERYTHROPOIESIS

The major morphologic changes that occur during maturation of erythroid elements involve

1. A **reduction in cell size** with increasing cellular maturity.
2. A **change in cytoplasmic coloration** from basophilia in the most immature cells to an admixture of basophilia and eosinophilia in cells of intermediate maturity to complete cytoplasmic eosinophilia in the most mature cells in the series.
3. **Increasing condensation of nuclear chromatin** as cellular maturation proceeds, with eventual expulsion of the nucleus from the cell.

During maturation of erythroid cells, granules never appear in the cytoplasm, nor does the shape of the nucleus change from a round or slightly oval shape.

The earliest recognizable and largest cell (17–19 μm) in the erythroid series is the **proerythroblast.** The **nucleus** of the cell, which occupies the greater proportion of the cell volume, is **slightly condensed,** and the cell exhibits **moderately basophilic cytoplasm.**

The proerythroblast gives rise to the **basophilic erythroblast,** a smaller cell (12–16 μm) characterized by **deeply basophilic cytoplasm** and more condensed nuclear chromatin.

Basophilic erythroblasts give rise to the **polychromatophilic erythroblast,** a smaller cell (9–17 μm) with **markedly condensed nuclear chromatin** and **grayish pink cytoplasm** that reflects an admixture of basic and acidic dye uptake.

The polychromatophilic erythroblast gives rise to the **orthochromatophilic erythroblast,** whose size (8–10 μm) approximates that of mature anucleate erythrocytes. The **orthochromatophilic erythroblast** exhibits **markedly condensed (pyknotic) nuclear chromatin** and **pink to orange cytoplasm,** which most closely **reflects** the **color** of **mature erythrocytes** in the immediately surrounding area. Orthochromatic erythroblasts are amitotic and eventually extrude their nuclei. They differentiate into reticulocytes (see Chapter 8, Figure 8-8), which mature into circulating erythrocytes.

The different stages in the development of cells in the erythroid series are illustrated in Figures 9-6– 9-9.

MEGAKARYOPOIESIS

The megakaryocyte, from which platelets are derived, is by far the largest and most easily recognizable cell in bone marrow. The cell, ranging in diameter from 35 to 150 μm, has a unique multilobed nucleus that is the result of endomitosis. The megakaryoblast, which is the precursor of the megakaryocyte, is a surprisingly smaller cell, approximately 30–45 μm in diameter, with a bilobed nucleus and a moderately basophilic cytoplasm. Megakaryoblasts are extremely difficult to find in normal marrow, whereas megakaryocytes, once identified, are rarely forgotten. An example of a megakaryoblast is shown in Figure 9-10; maturing megakaryocytes are shown in Figures 9-11– 9-13.

MONOCYTOPOIESIS

The earliest precursor to monocytes is difficult to distinguish from other blast cells in normal marrow. The cell gives rise to a promonocyte (Figure 9-16), which is 16–18 μm in diameter and has a slightly indented nucleus and slate gray cytoplasm that may or may not display fine azurophilic granulation. Promonocytes give rise to mature monocytes that range in size from 11–18 μm in diameter, have a distinctive indented or kidney-shaped nucleus, and in well-fixed and stained preparations, display fine azurophilic granulation in their cytoplasm (see Chapter 8, Figures 8-1 and 8-6).

LYMPHOPOIESIS

Whereas lymphocytes are produced primarily in lymphatic tissue, lymphocyte precursors are produced in marrow. Bone marrow stem cells continually seed lymphatic tissue, in particular the thymus, and there give rise to lymphocytes indigenous to the particular tissue. In marrow under normal conditions, lymphoblasts and prolymphocytes are rarely encountered. Small lymphocytes, however, can be found and are often mistaken for late polychromatophilic or early orthochromatophilic erythroblasts because of their similar size and sometimes similar cytoplasmic staining. Small lymphocytes (Figures 9-2 and 9-16) are distinguished from erythroid elements by their less clumped nuclei, which may be slightly indented, and thin rim of lightly basophilic cytoplasm.

In addition to the aforementioned cells, plasma cells are observed in normal marrow. Although plasmablasts and proplasmacytes are rarely seen in normal marrow, the mature plasma cell has a distinctive morphology (Figure 9-17). The plasma cell is characterized by an eccentrically placed nucleus with moderate to densely clumped chromatin (cartwheel shaped), a clear perinuclear area, and moderately to deeply basophilic-staining cytoplasm.

FIGURE 9-1
Photomicrograph illustrating a promyelocyte (1), myelocyte (2), metamyelocyte (4), band (5), and segmented cell of the developing neutrophilic series (6). Oe, orthochromatophilic erythroblast; N, nucleolus. Wright's stain. × 1376.

FIGURE 9-2
Photomicrograph depicting a myeloblast (MB), early neutrophilic myelocytes (2), late neutrophilic myelocytes (3), neutrophilic metamyelocytes (4), band neutrophils (5), and a mature neutrophil (6). Note the polar view of an unidentifiable bone marrow cell (arrow) in the metaphase stage of mitosis, the small lymphocyte (L), and orthochromatophilic erythroblast (Oe). N, nucleolus. Wright's stain. × 1376.

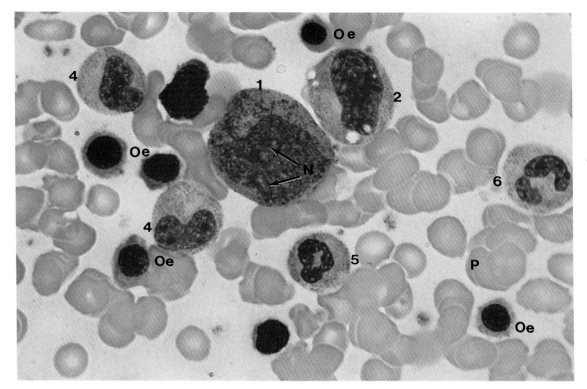

figure 9-1

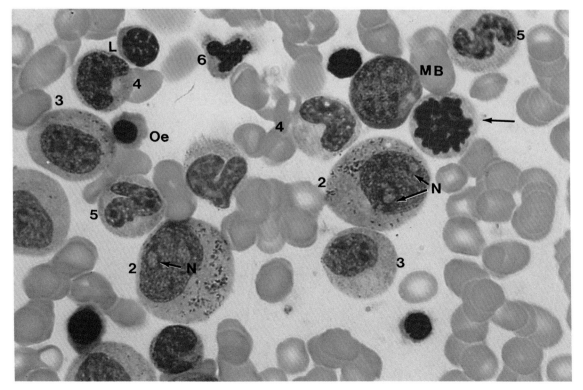

figure 9-2

FIGURE 9-3
Photomicrograph illustrating a neutrophilic myelocyte (3), neutrophilic metamyelocytes (4), a band neutrophil (5), and a segmented neutrophil (6). Note the orthochromatophilic erythroblasts (Oe). Wright's stain. × 1376.

FIGURE 9-4
Photomicrograph contrasting an eosinophilic myelocyte (EM) with two neutrophilic myelocytes (3), a neutrophilic metamyelocyte (4), and a band neutrophil (5). Oe, orthochromatophilic erythroblast. Wright's stain. × 1376.

FIGURE 9-5
Photomicrograph of an eosinophilic metamyelocyte (EMm) and a mature neutrophil (6). Compare the eosinophilic metamyelocyte with the neutrophilic metamyelocytes in Figures 9-1–9-4. Wright's stain. × 1376.

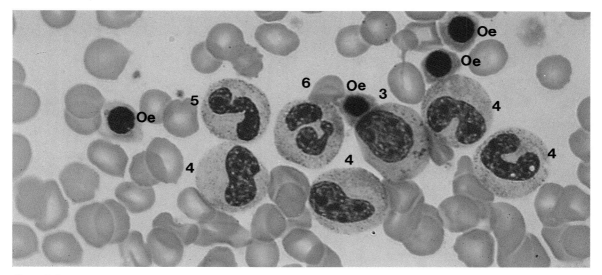

figure 9-3

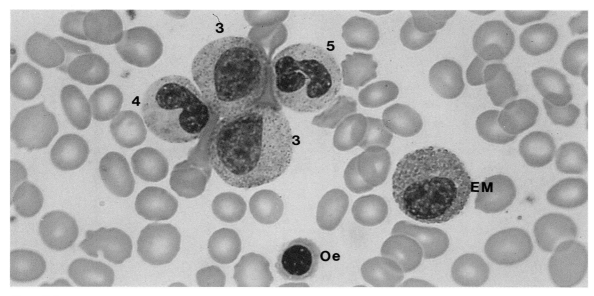

figure 9-4

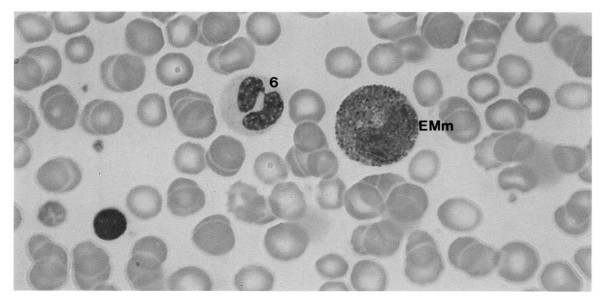

figure 9-5

FIGURE 9-6

Photomicrograph of the earliest recognizable cell, the proerythroblast (P), of the erythroid cell series. Also shown are a neutrophilic myelocyte (3), neutrophilic meta-myelocyte (4), band neutrophil (5), and mature neutrophil (6). Wright's stain. × 1376.

FIGURE 9-7

Photomicrograph that contrasts the morphology of a basophilic erythroblast (B) with that of a promyelocyte (1) and a neutrophilic myelocyte (3). Compare both the basophilic erythroblast and promyelocyte with the proerythroblast in Figure 9-6. OE, ortho-chromatophilic erythroblast; 5, band neutrophil. Wright's stain. × 1376.

FIGURE 9-8

Photomicrograph illustrating two polychromatophilic erythroblasts (Pe), a late polychromatophilic erythroblast (LPe), and an orthochromatophilic erythroblast (Oe). Wright's stain. × 1376.

FIGURE 9-9

Photomicrograph of polychromatophilic (Pe), late polychromatophilic (LPe), and ortho-chromatophilic (Oe) erythroblasts. Also shown are an eosinophilic myelocyte (EM), a late neutrophilic myelocyte (3), and a band neutrophil (5). Wright's stain. × 1376.

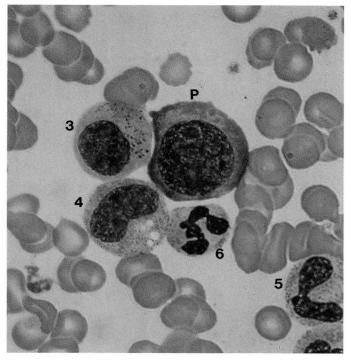

figure 9-6

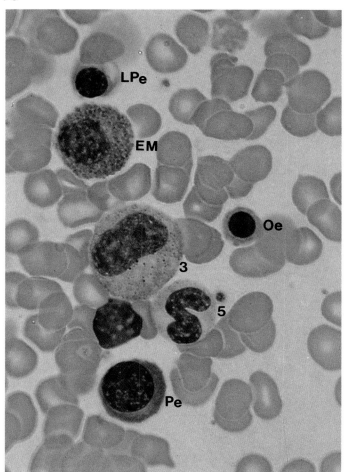

figure 9-7

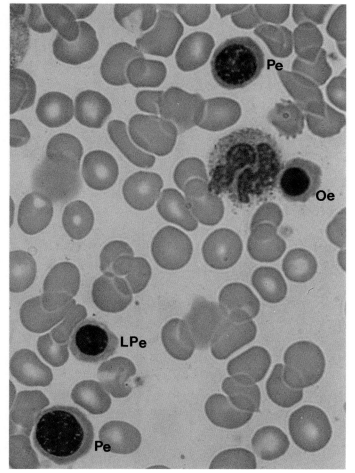

figure 9-8

figure 9-9

FIGURE 9-10
Photomicrograph illustrating a megakaryocytoblast (arrow). Note the bilobed nucleus and faintly basophilic cytoplasm of the cell. 3, Neutrophilic myelocyte; 4, neutrophilic metamyelocytes. Wright's stain. × 1376.

FIGURE 9-11
Photomicrograph of an immature megakaryocyte. Lobulation of the nucleus is not readily distinguished. Wright's stain. × 1032.

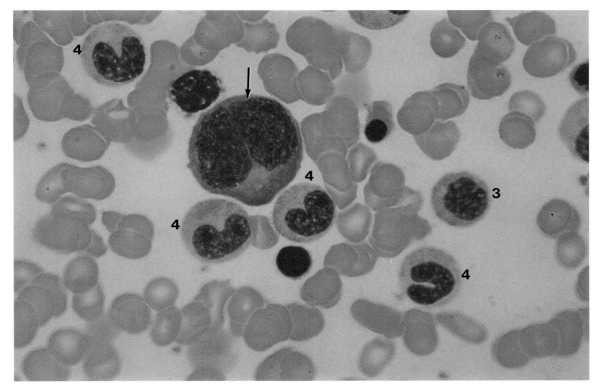

figure 9-10

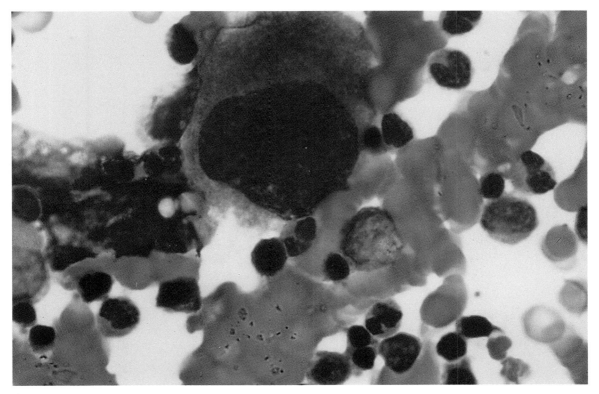

figure 9-11

FIGURE 9-12
Photomicrograph of a megakaryocyte displaying a multilobulated nucleus and granular-appearing cytoplasm. Wright's stain. × 1032.

FIGURE 9-13
Photomicrograph of a mature megakaryocyte. Wright's stain. × 1032.

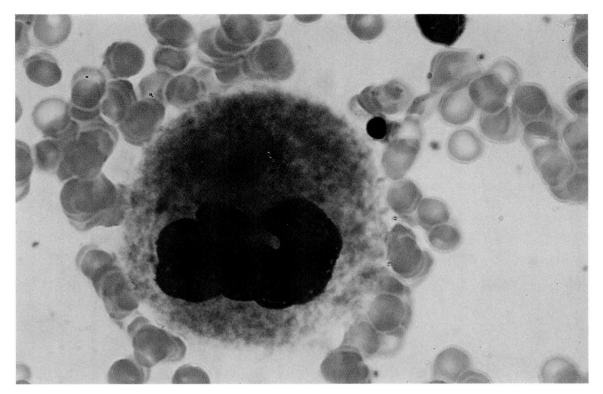

figure 9-12

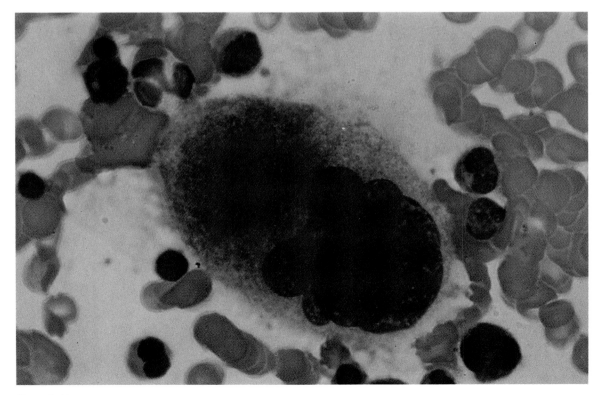

figure 9-13

FIGURE 9-14

Electron micrograph of part of a mature megakaryocyte. The multilobed nucleus presents a bizarre profile. Note the demarcation vesicles (D) and granules (G) in the cytoplasm. Mouse marrow; × 9300.

FIGURE 9-15

Electron micrograph of a part of the peripheral cytoplasm of a megakaryocyte showing the granulomere (G), demarcation vesicles (D), and a blebbing of the hyalomere (H). P, platelet. Mouse marrow; × 36,000.

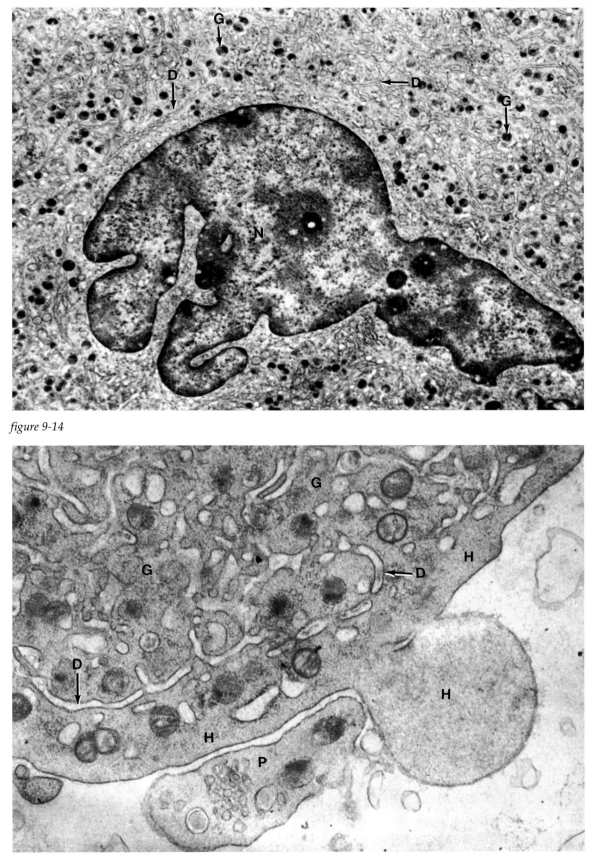

figure 9-14

figure 9-15

FIGURE 9-16
Photomicrograph of a promonocyte (PM), neutrophilic metamyelocyte (4), and band neutrophil (5). Note the small lymphocyte (L). Wright's stain. × 1376.

FIGURE 9-17
Photomicrograph illustrating a plasma cell (PL), late polychromatophilic erythroblast (LPe), two orthochromatophilic erythroblasts (Oe), a neutrophilic myelocyte (3), and two band neutrophils (5). Wright's stain. × 1376.

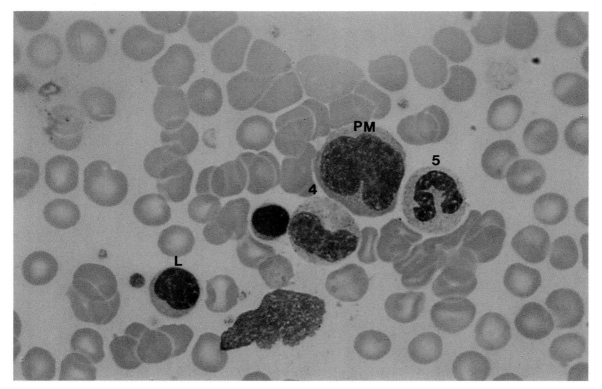

figure 9-16

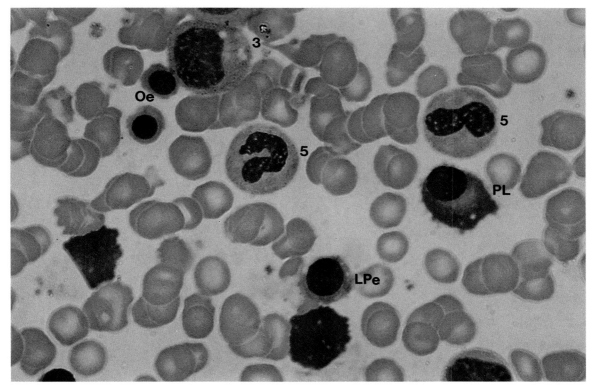

figure 9-17

FIGURE 9-18
Photomicrograph of a basophilic erythroblast in very late telophase of mitosis. Wright's stain. × 1376.

FIGURE 9-19
Photomicrograph showing a polychromatophilic erythroblast (arrow) in mitosis. Also apparent are a polychromatophilic erythroblast (Pe), late polychromatophilic erythroblast (LPe), early neutrophilic myelocyte (2), late neutrophilic myelocyte (3), and band neutrophil (5). Wright's stain. × 1376.

FIGURE 9-20
Photomicrograph of two polychromatophilic erythroblasts just prior to completion of cytokinesis. Wright's stain. × 1376.

FIGURE 9-21
Photomicrograph of a polar view of a neutrophilic myelocyte (arrow) in metaphase of mitosis. Also apparent are a monocyte (M), late neutrophilic myelocytes (3), a neutrophilic metamyelocyte (4), and band neutrophils (5). Wright's stain. × 1376.

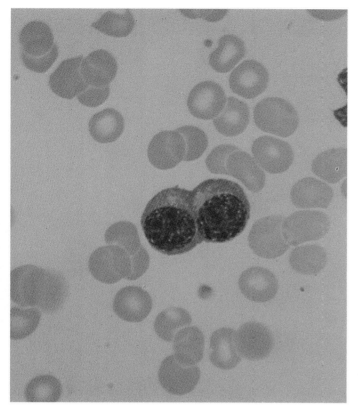

figure 9-18

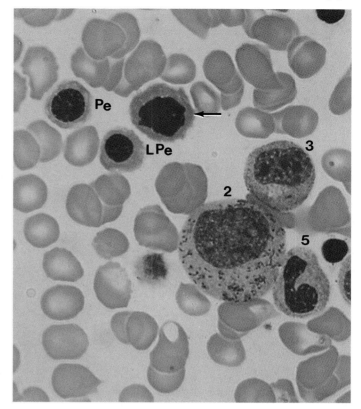

figure 9-19

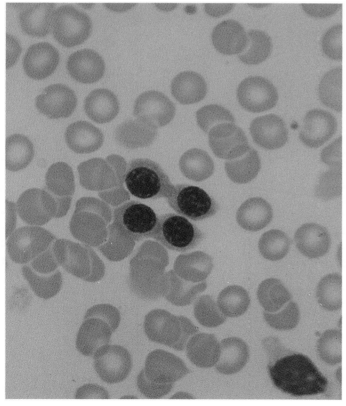

figure 9-20

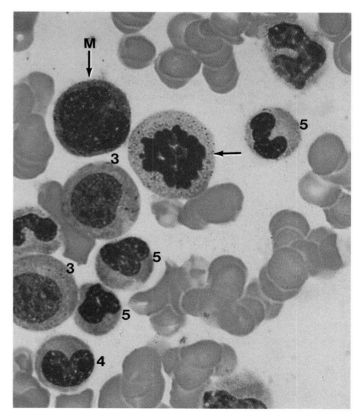

figure 9-21

10 Lymphoid System

FIGURE 10-1

Photomicrograph of the smallest functioning unit of the lymphoid system, the small lymphocyte, as seen in a smear preparation of peripheral blood. Wright's stain. × 1376.

FIGURE 10-2

Photomicrograph illustrating lymphocyte infiltration (arrows) in the epithelium and lamina propria of a small intestinal villus. Note the central lacteal (C), a lymphatic capillary, its endothelial lining cells (E), and lymphocytes within the lumen of the lacteal. The nucleus (N) of what appears to be a neutrophilic leukocyte is seen in the lamina propria. × 560.

FIGURE 10-3

Photomicrograph of diffuse lymphatic tissue (arrows) in loose connective tissue. Note the difference in the nuclear shapes of the lymphocytes and fibroblasts (F). × 560.

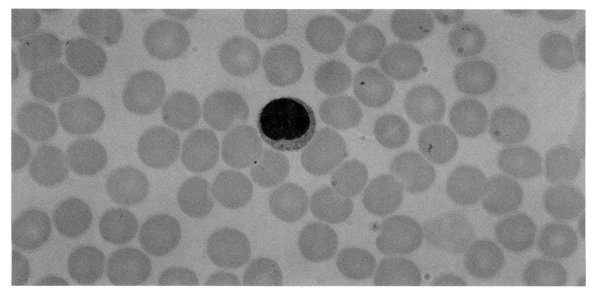

figure 10-1

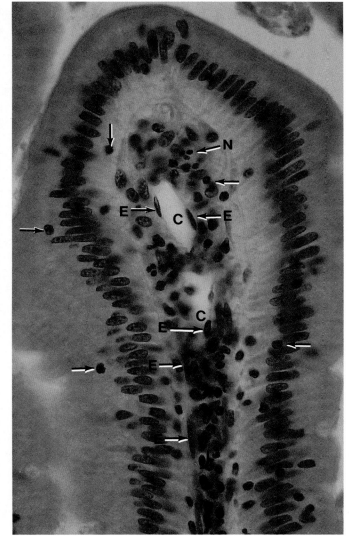

figure 10-2

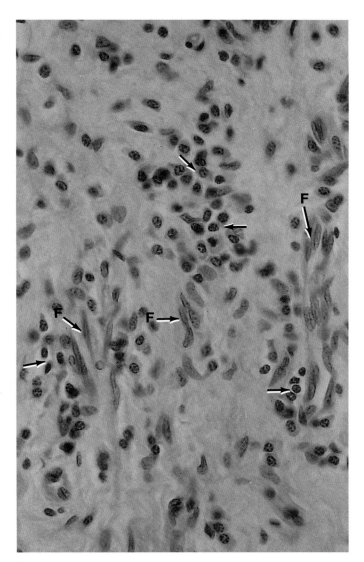

figure 10-3

FIGURE 10-4

Photomicrograph of a small nodular aggregate of lymphocytes with two cells in mitosis (arrows). × 560.

FIGURE 10-5

Photomicrograph depicting nodular aggregates of lymphocytes (N), Peyer's patches, in the ileum. The pale staining region (arrow) in two of the nodules is called the germinal center, and the nodule is called a secondary nodule. × 56.

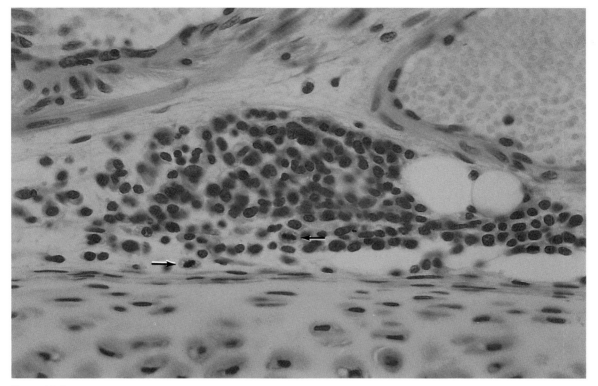

figure 10-4

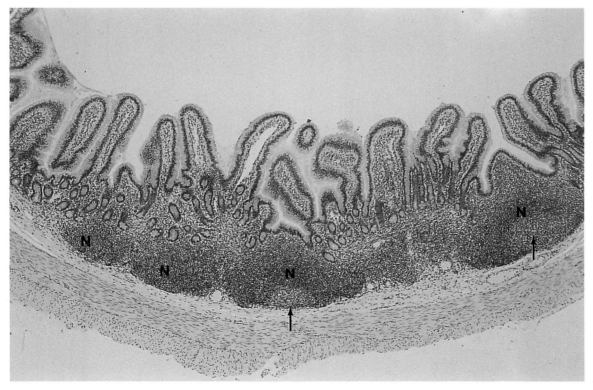

figure 10-5

FIGURE 10-6

Photomicrograph of a germinal center (G) of a secondary nodule. Note the mitotic figures (arrows) in the germinal center and the mantle zone (M) of the nodule. × 344.

FIGURE 10-7

Photomicrograph emphasizing the morphologic difference between the mantle zone and pale-staining germinal center of a secondary nodule. Note the large pale-staining nuclei of cells in the germinal center (arrows), in contrast to the small dense-staining nuclei of cells in the mantle zone (M). × 560.

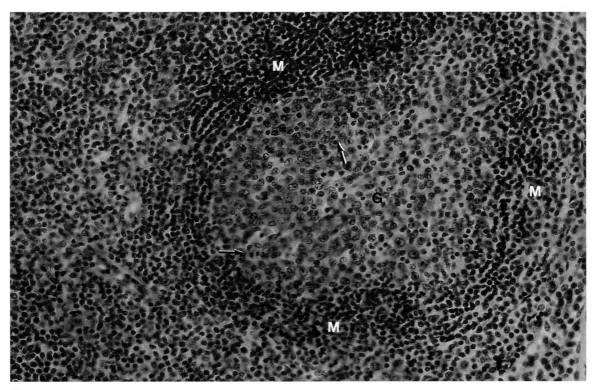

figure 10-6

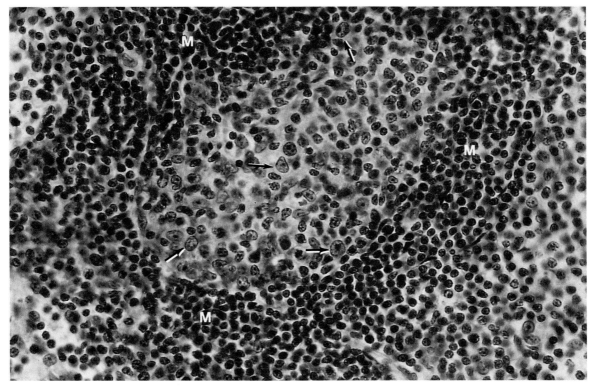

figure 10-7

FIGURE 10-8
Photomicrograph of the appendix illustrating the abundant concentration of lympho-cytes (L), the dark staining material in the mucosa and submucosa of the organ. × 56.

FIGURE 10-9
Photomicrograph of the large intestine depicting a secondary lymphatic nodule with a well-developed germinal center (G). × 56.

FIGURE 10-10
Photomicrograph of palatine tonsil, a partially encapsulated lymphoid organ illustrat-ing a multiplicity of secondary lymphatic nodules with prominent germinal centers (G). Note the stratified squamous epithelium (arrows) and epithelial invaginations that form crypts (C). CA, connective tissue of the capsule; S, connective tissue of the septum. × 56.

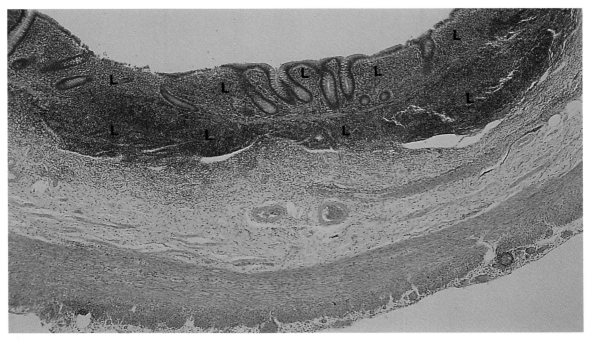

figure 10-8

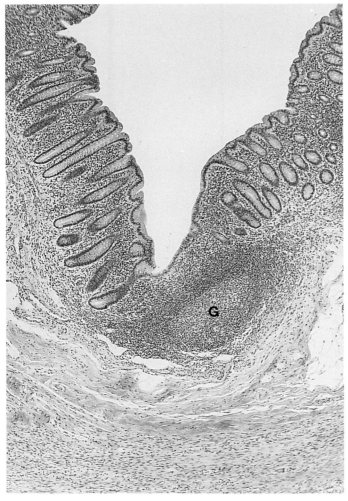

figure 10-9

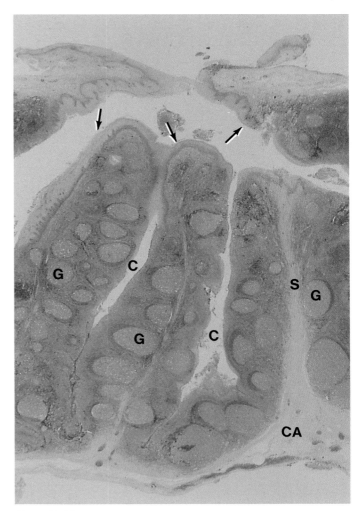

figure 10-10

FIGURE 10-11

Photomicrograph of a whole lymph node illustrating the morphology of its major regions, the cortex (Co), paracortex (Pc), medulla (M), and hilum (H). Note the faintly stained capsule (arrows), which is more clearly seen in Figure 10-14, germinal centers of secondary nodules (G) in the cortex, and medullary cords of lymphocytes (Mc). × 56.

FIGURE 10-12

Scanning electron micrograph illustrating the organization of the cortex of a lymph node. Depicted is part of the connective tissue capsule (Ca) and two lymph nodules (LN). Blood vessels (BV) are apparent, as are branching cell processes (arrows) of reticular cells in the subcapsular (SS) and cortical (CS) sinuses. × 1145. (Reprinted with permission from *Tissue and Organs: A Text-Atlas of Scanning Electron Microscopy*, by Richard G. Kessel and Randy H. Kardon. Copyright © 1979 W. H. Freeman & Company.)

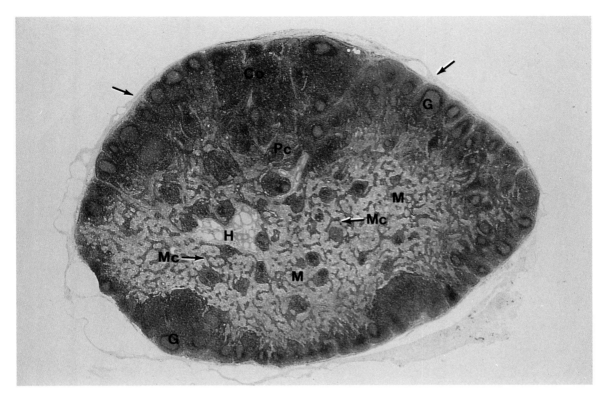

figure 10-11

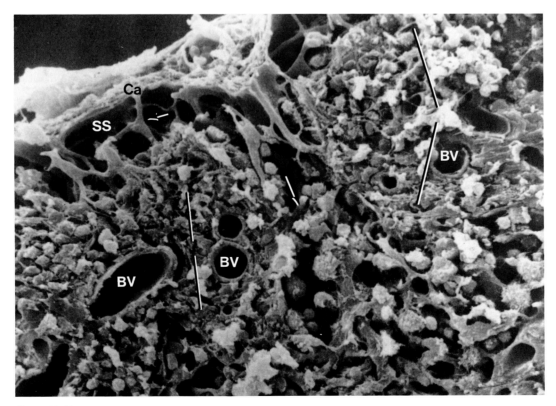

figure 10-12

FIGURE 10-13

Photomicrograph of the cortex of a lymph node illustrating its capsule (C), subcapsular sinus (Ss), connective tissue trabecula (T), trabecula sinus (Ts), and germinal centers of secondary nodules in the cortex (G). Pc, paracortex. × 56.

FIGURE 10-14

Photomicrograph of the medulla of a lymph node depicting medullary sinuses (Ms), medullary cords of lymphocytes (arrows), and blood vessels (V). × 140.

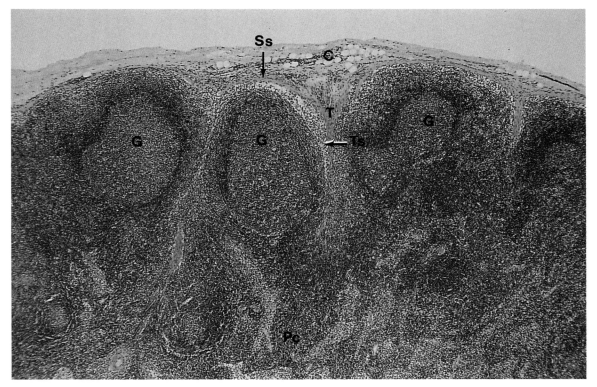

figure 10-13

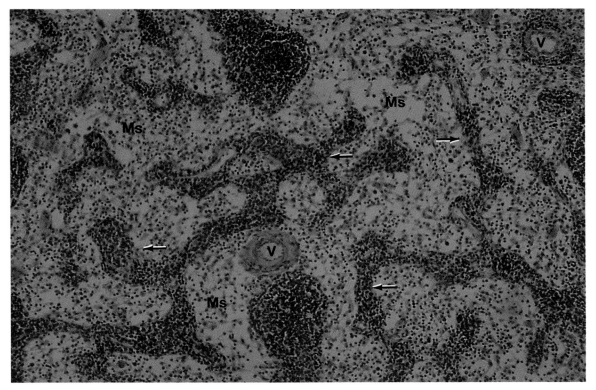

figure 10-14

FIGURE 10-15

Photomicrograph of the cortex of a lymph node depicting the connective tissue capsule (C) and trabecula (T) of the external nodal framework and blue-staining reticular fibers of the internal framework. Note the paucity of reticular fibers in the lymphatic nodules (N) in comparison with their concentration in the paracortical (Pc) and internodular regions. Co, cortex. Silver stain. × 140.

FIGURE 10-16

Photomicrograph illustrating the delicate meshwork of reticular fibers (arrows) in the medulla of a lymph node. V, blood vessel. Silver stain. × 344.

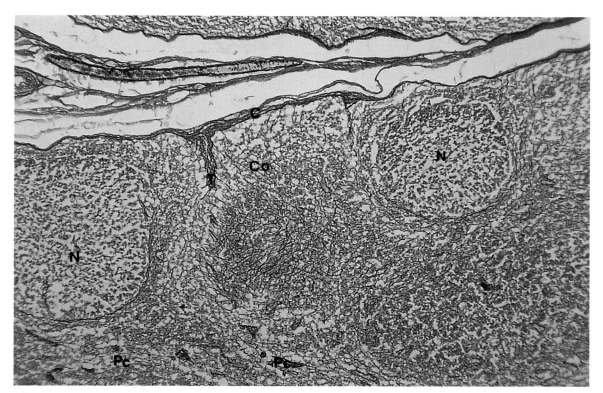

figure 10-15

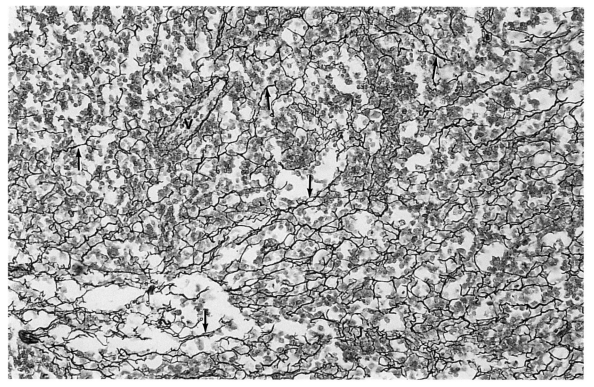

figure 10-16

FIGURE 10-17

Photomicrograph illustrating the lymphatic nodules (N) of the white pulp and areas of red pulp (R) of the spleen. Note the blood vessel, the central artery (arrows), within nodules that is specific to the white pulp and the spleen. Also illustrated are the splenic connective tissue capsule (C) and trabeculae (T) of connective tissue, which contain blood vessels (V) and incompletely compartmentalize the organ. G, germinal center. × 56.

FIGURE 10-18

Photomicrograph of a secondary splenic nodule (N) and adjacent surrounding red pulp (R). Note the periarteriolar lymphatic sheath (PALS), made up of lymphocytes that immediately surround a central artery (arrow). G, germinal center of the secondary nodule. × 140.

FIGURE 10-19

Scanning electron micrograph of a cast of part of the vasculature within a splenic nodule. The cellular elements of the white pulp (WP), in particular the periarteriolar lymphatic sheath that surrounds the central artery (CA), have been removed by digestion with an alkaline solution. Note how the branches of the central artery, the follicular arterioles (FA), arborize in the white pulp and terminate in marginal sinuses (MS). × 170. (Reprinted with permission from *Tissue and Organs: A Text-Atlas of Scanning Electron Microscopy*, by Richard G. Kessel and Randy H. Kardon. Copyright © 1979 W. H. Freeman & Company.)

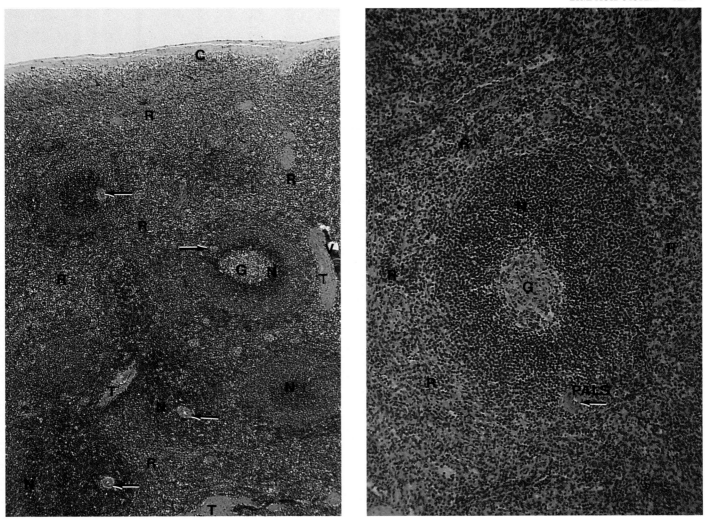

figure 10-17

figure 10-18

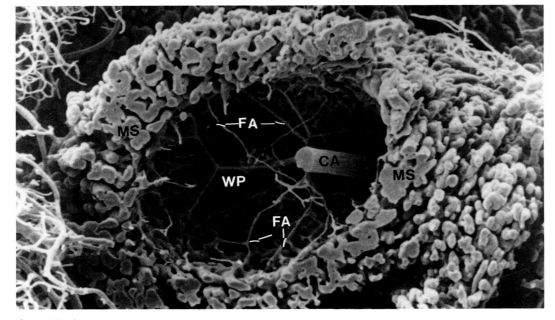

figure 10-19

FIGURE 10-20
Photomicrograph of a portion of red and white pulp of the spleen. The central artery (arrow) of the nodule in the white pulp is surrounded by lymphocytes of the periarteriolar lymphatic sheath (PALS). Note the difference in concentration of lymphocytes in the PALS and the marginal zone (MZ) of the nodule. The splenic red pulp is made up of sinusoids (S) and intervening cellular elements, the cords of Billroth (C). × 344.

FIGURE 10-21
Photomicrograph of splenic red pulp. S, sinuses; C, cords of Billroth. × 560.

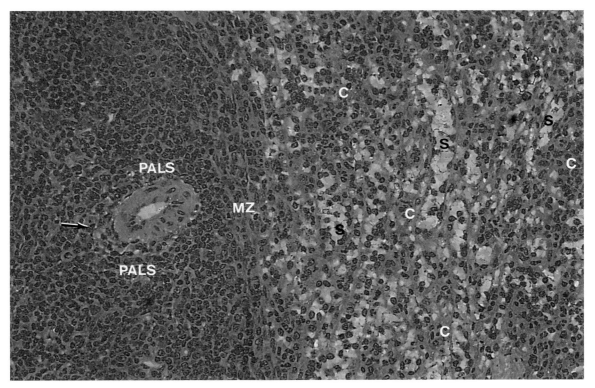

figure 10-20

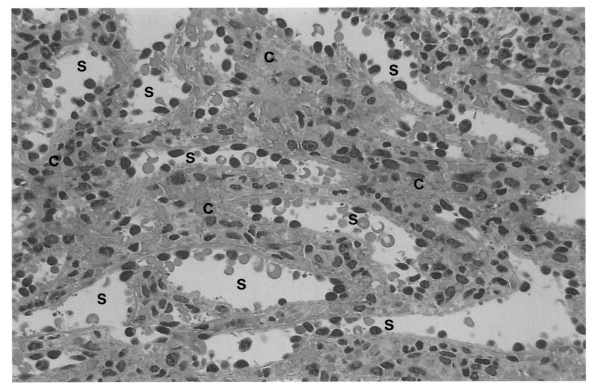

figure 10-21

FIGURE 10-22

Photomicrograph of a portion of the thymus. Note the absence of nodular aggregates in the cortex (C) and medulla (M) and the difference in lymphocyte (thymocyte) concentration in these regions of the gland. A thymic or Hassall's corpuscle (arrow) is seen in the medulla. CT, connective tissue. × 140.

FIGURE 10-23

Photomicrograph of epithelial reticular cells (arrows) and small lymphocytes (thymocytes) of the thymus. × 869.

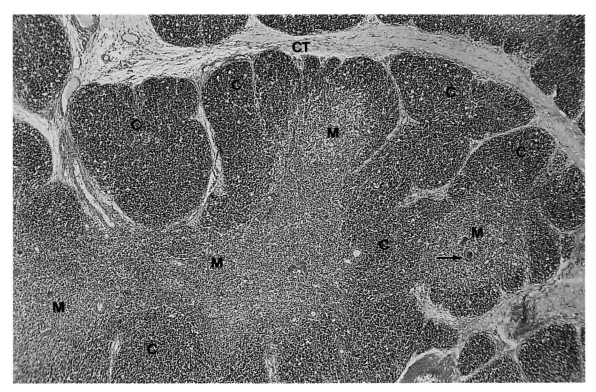

figure 10-22

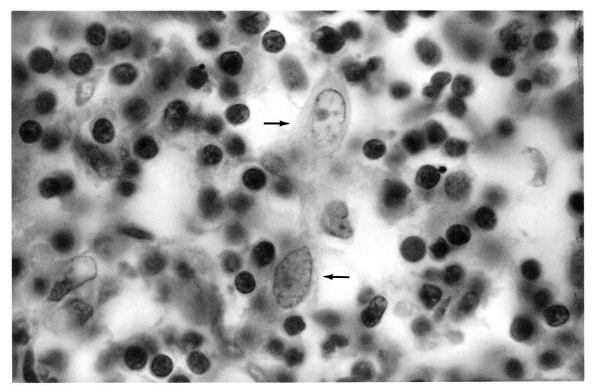

figure 10-23

FIGURE 10-24
Photomicrograph illustrating central cellular degeneration and the concentric arrangement of epithelial reticular cells that comprise a thymic, or Hassall's, corpuscle (H). Also seen are epithelial reticular cells of the medulla (arrows). × 560.

FIGURE 10-25
Photomicrograph depicting hyalinization of epithelial reticular cells in a thymic corpuscle (H) and epithelial reticular cells (arrows) of the medulla. × 560.

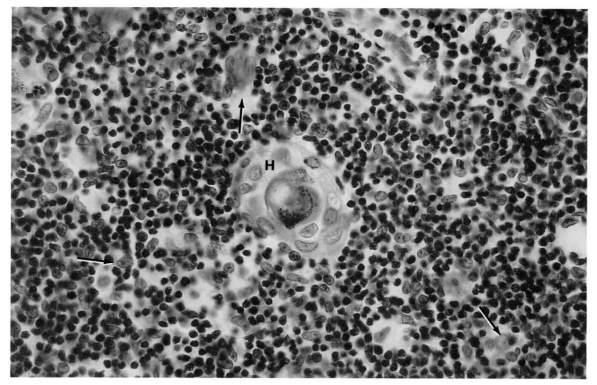

figure 10-24

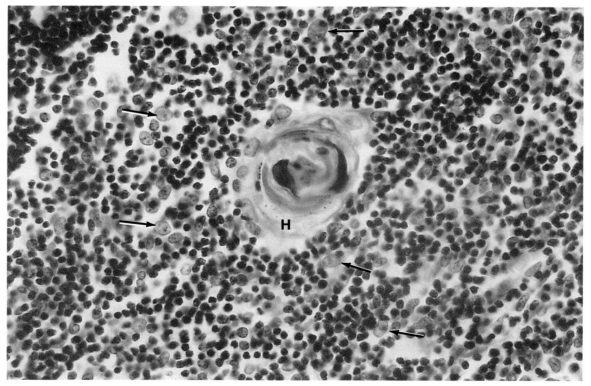

figure 10-25

11 Circulatory System

FIGURE 11-1

Scanning electron micrograph of a blood vessel illustrating three basic structural features (tunics) that to varying degrees are common to all parts of the circulatory system. In blood vessels, the layer closest to the lumen (Lu), the tunica intima (TI), is composed of a single layer of endothelial cells (EC) supported by connective tissue. In the heart, this tunic is called the endocardium. The tunica media (TM), or middle layer, is composed chiefly of smooth muscle (except in the aorta). In the heart, this layer is called the myocardium. External to the tunica media is the tunica adventitia (TA), a connective tissue layer, which in the heart corresponds to the epicardium. × 3915. (Reprinted with permission from *Tissue and Organs: A Text-Atlas of Scanning Electron Microscopy*, by Richard G. Kessel and Randy H. Kardon. Copyright © 1979 W. H. Freeman & Company.)

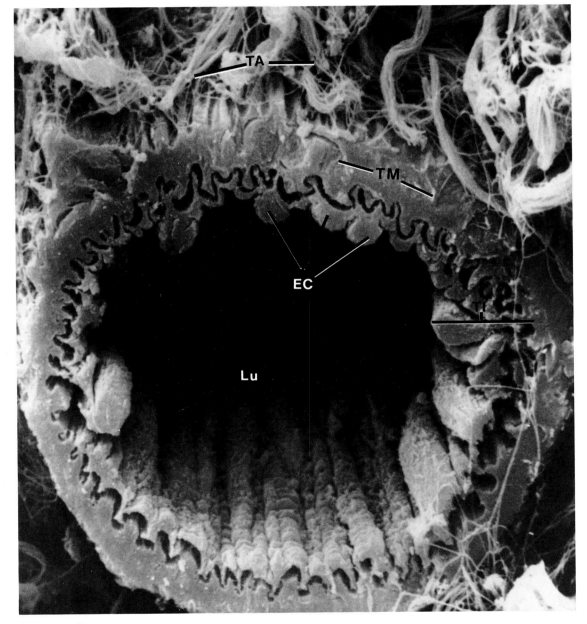

figure 11-1

FIGURE 11-13

Low-power photomicrograph illustrating a medium (muscular) artery (MA), a medium (muscular) vein (MV), a small artery (A), a small vein (V), a nerve bundle (N), and fat (F). Elastic stain. × 49.

FIGURE 11-14

Higher-power photomicrograph of part of the muscular artery shown in Figure 11-13. Note the prominent internal elastic lamina (IEL) and external elastic lamina (EEL), which delimit the tunica intima (I) from the smooth muscle (Sm) of the tunica media (M) and the tunica media from the connective tissue of the tunica adventitia (A), respectively. Note the paucity of elastic fibers in the tunica media. Elastic stain. × 122.

FIGURE 11-15

Higher-power magnification of part of the muscular vein shown in Figure 11-13. The tunica intima (I) is extremely thin and cannot be readily distinguished from the smooth muscle (Sm) of the tunica media (M). Note the well-developed tunica adventitia (A) and the nuclei of the endothelial cells (arrows) of the tunica intima. Elastic stain. × 122.

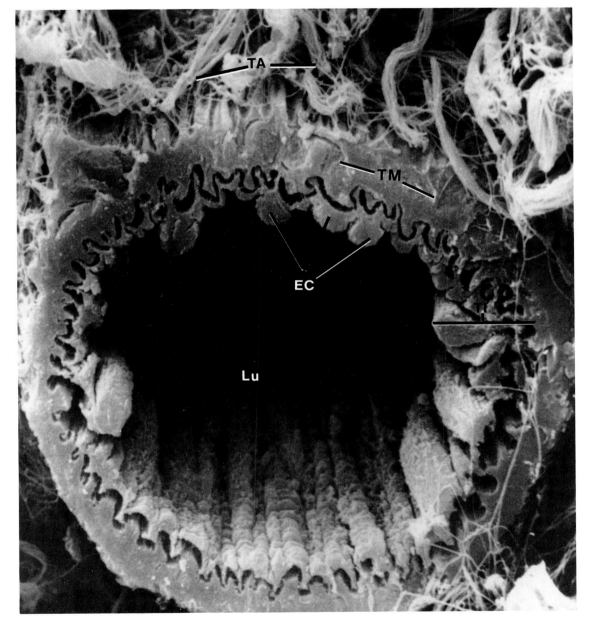

figure 11-1

FIGURE 11-2

Photomicrograph of the left atrioventricular valve illustrating the continuity of the valve leaflet (arrow) with the endocardium (En) of the atrium (A). In this preparation, collagen (C) is stained green. Note that the connective tissue of the endocardium and that of the valve are not entirely collagenous. M, myocardium; CT, chordae tendineae; A, atrium; V, ventricle. Masson's stain. × 14.

FIGURE 11-3

Higher magnification of a part of the atrioventricular valve depicted in Figure 11-2. Note the endothelial covering on both surfaces of the valve and uneven distribution of collagen (C) in the core of the valve. Elastic fibers (EL) are prominent directly beneath the endothelium (E). CT, chordae tendineae. Masson's stain. × 56.

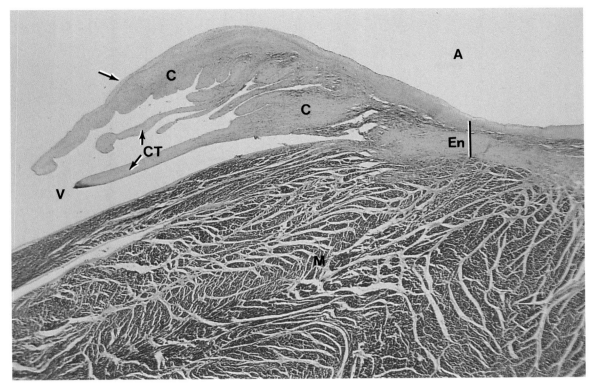

figure 11-2

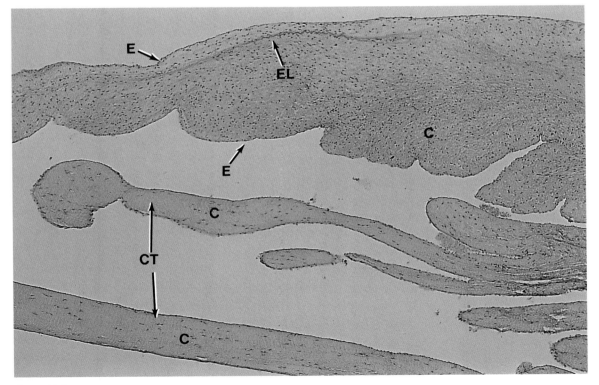

figure 11-3

FIGURE 11-4

Photomicrograph depicting trabeculae carneae (ventricular folds). Note the thin endocardium (En) of the ventricle. M, myocardium. × 56.

FIGURE 11-5

Photomicrograph depicting the epicardium (Ep) of a ventricle. Note the nerve bundle (N) in the connective tissue of the epicardium. A remnant of the mesothelium that covers the epicardium is seen at the arrow. M, myocardium. × 56.

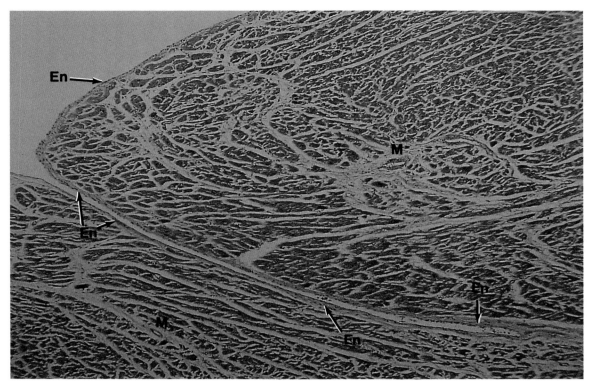

figure 11-4

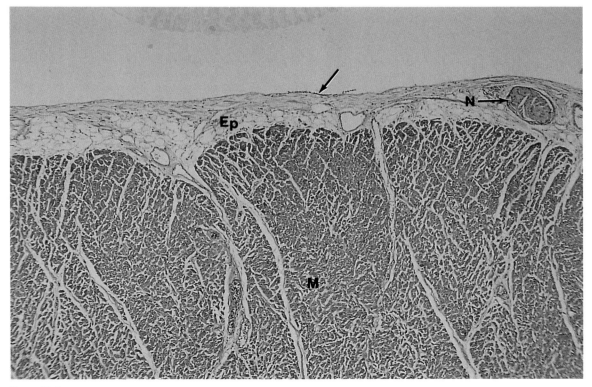

figure 11-5

FIGURE 11-6
Photomicrograph of the endocardium (En) of the atrium. Note the thick subendothelial connective tissue (CT). E, endothelium; M, myocardium. × 140.

FIGURE 11-7
Photomicrograph of the epicardium (Ep) of the atrium. Note the mesothelial cell covering (arrows), nerve bundle (N), and fat (F) of the epicardium. CT, connective tissue; M, myocardium. × 140.

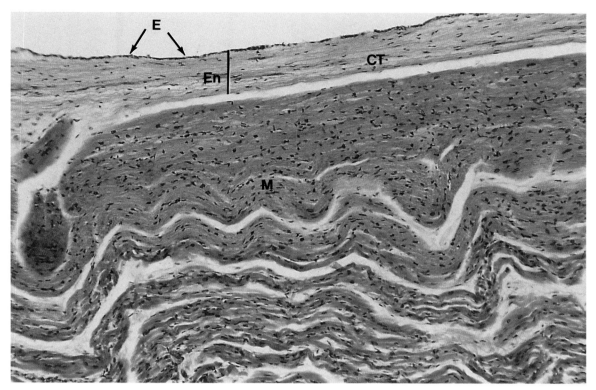

figure 11-6

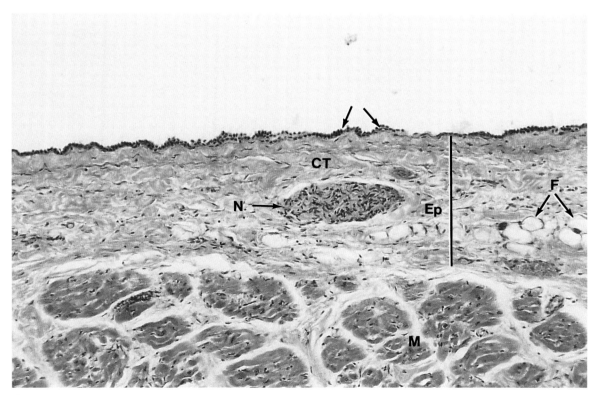

figure 11-7

FIGURE 11-8

Photomicrograph of the endocardium (En) of an atrium stained with Masson's tri-chrome stain. Note the simple squamous cells of the endothelium (E). There is a paucity of collagen (C) directly beneath the endothelium, a region with a preponderance of elastic and reticular fibers over collagen fibers. M, myocardium; I, intercalated disc. × 344.

FIGURE 11-9

Photomicrograph depicting Purkinje fibers (PF) in the subendothelial connective tissue (CT) of an atrium. M, myocardium (M). Beef heart; × 140.

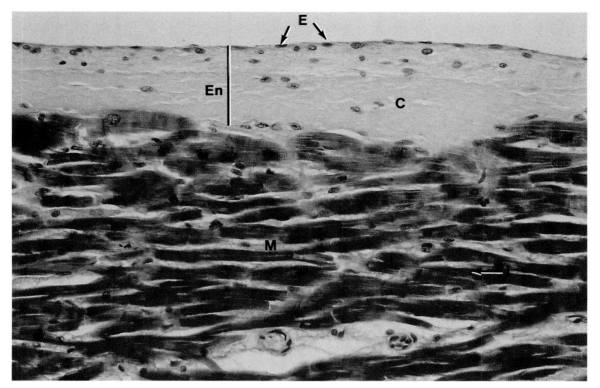

figure 11-8

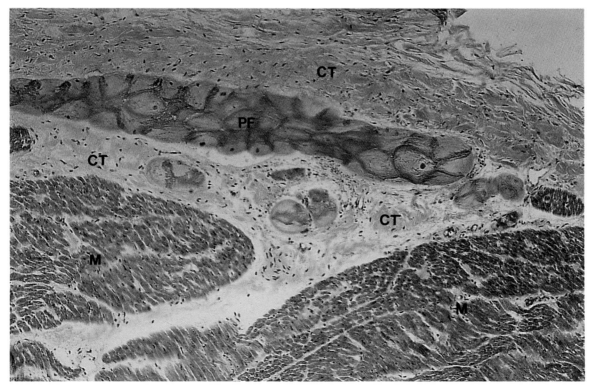

figure 11-9

FIGURE 11-10

Photomicrograph illustrating the morphologic features of the aorta, a large elastic artery. Note in particular the width of the tunica media (M) in contrast to the width of the tunica intima (I) and tunica adventitia (A). Elastic stain. × 49.

FIGURE 11-11

Higher magnification of part of the aorta shown in Figure 11-10, emphasizing the density of elastic fibers in the thick tunica media (M), which constitutes the greater part of the vessel wall. The internal elastic lamina (IEL) demarcates the tunica intima (I) from the tunica media. Note the vasa vasora (V), blood vessels, and elastic fibers in the tunica adventitia (A). Arrows point to cells of the endothelium. Elastic stain. × 122.

FIGURE 11-12

Photomicrograph of a large vein, the inferior vena cava, stained for elastic fibers. The tunica media (M), which occupies a lesser proportion of the vessel wall than does the tunica media of the aorta, consists primarily of smooth muscle, with some elastic fibers (EF). A prominent internal elastic lamina (IEL) delimits the well-developed tunica intima (I) from the tunica media. Arrows point to endothelial cells of the tunica intima. A, tunica adventitia. Elastic stain. × 122.

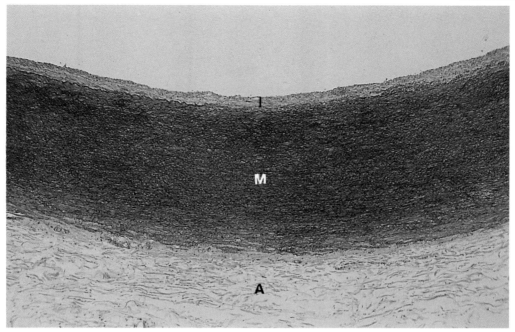

figure 11-10

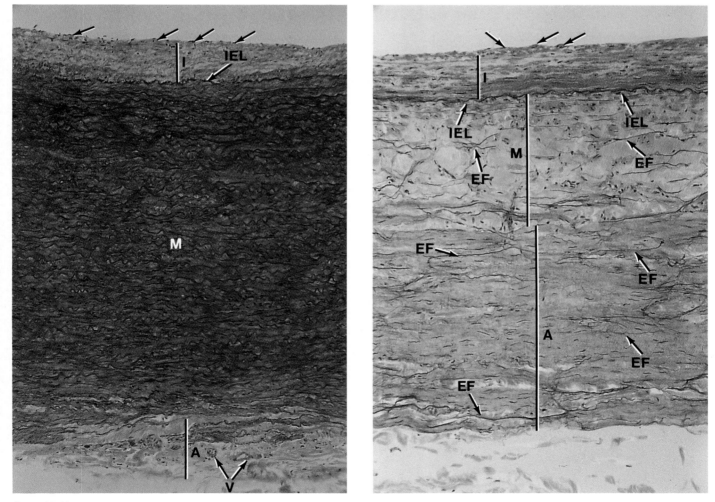

figure 11-11

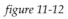

figure 11-12

FIGURE 11-13

Low-power photomicrograph illustrating a medium (muscular) artery (MA), a medium (muscular) vein (MV), a small artery (A), a small vein (V), a nerve bundle (N), and fat (F). Elastic stain. × 49.

FIGURE 11-14

Higher-power photomicrograph of part of the muscular artery shown in Figure 11-13. Note the prominent internal elastic lamina (IEL) and external elastic lamina (EEL), which delimit the tunica intima (I) from the smooth muscle (Sm) of the tunica media (M) and the tunica media from the connective tissue of the tunica adventitia (A), respectively. Note the paucity of elastic fibers in the tunica media. Elastic stain. × 122.

FIGURE 11-15

Higher-power magnification of part of the muscular vein shown in Figure 11-13. The tunica intima (I) is extremely thin and cannot be readily distinguished from the smooth muscle (Sm) of the tunica media (M). Note the well-developed tunica adventitia (A) and the nuclei of the endothelial cells (arrows) of the tunica intima. Elastic stain. × 122.

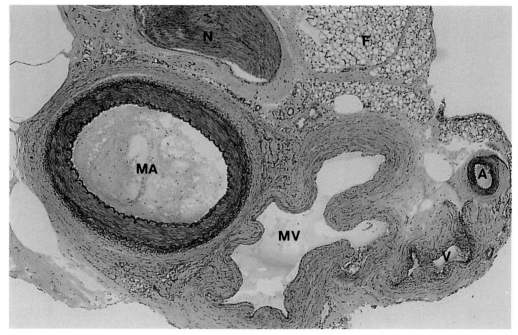

figure 11-13

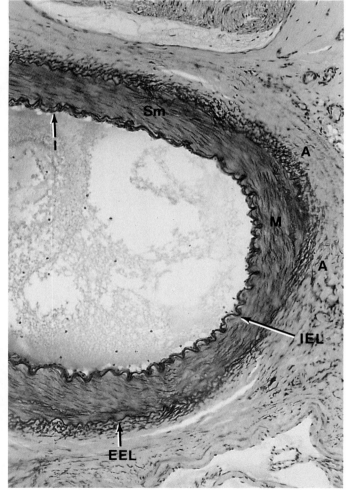

figure 11-14

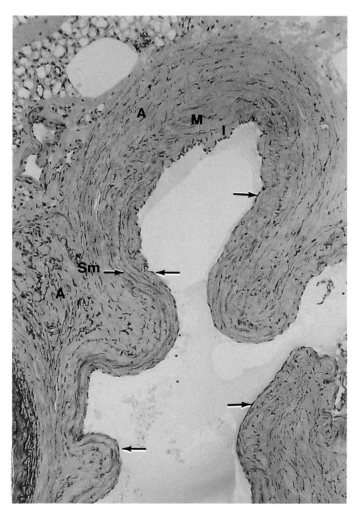

figure 11-15

FIGURE 11-16

Photomicrograph of a small artery (A) and small vein (V) in the tunica albuginea of the testis. Note the smooth muscle of the well-developed tunica media (M) of the artery and nuclei of endothelial cells (E; arrows). In the vein, the tunica media is poorly developed and cannot be distinguished from the tunica intima (unlabeled arrow). Both vessels have a prominent adventitia (Ad), which they share in common in the area labeled X. × 140.

FIGURE 11-17

Photomicrograph contrasting the morphology of a small artery and a small vein in the medulla of the kidney. The tunica media (M) and tunica adventitia (Ad) are readily identified in the artery (A), whereas all three tunics of the vein (V) are poorly demarcated. × 140.

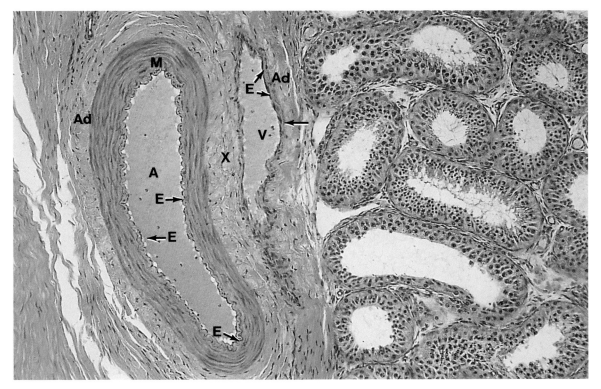

figure 11-16

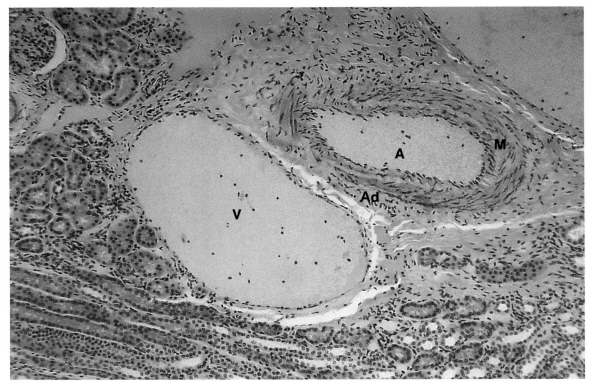

figure 11-17

FIGURE 11-18
Photomicrograph of a small vein with portions of two valve leaflets (arrow). × 140.

FIGURE 11-19
Photomicrograph of a small vein with a valve (arrow). Connective tissue, which is stained green in this preparation, forms the core of the valve. Both surfaces of the valve are lined by endothelial cells (arrows) that are continuous with the endothelium of the vessel's tunica intima. N, Nerve bundles. Masson's stain. × 140.

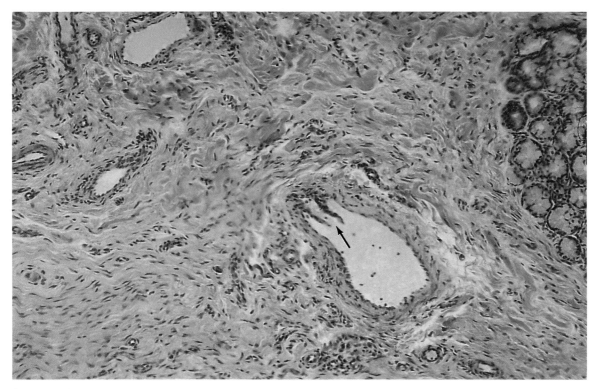

figure 11-18

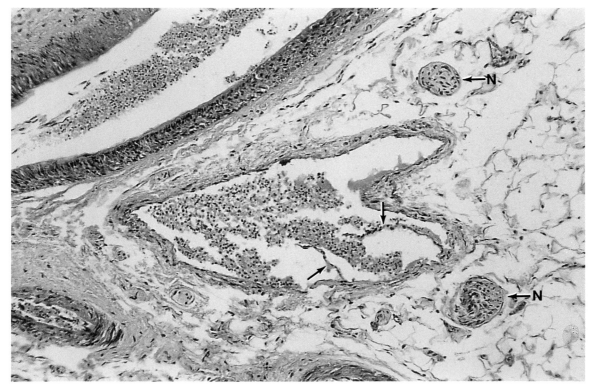

figure 11-19

FIGURE 11-20
Photomicrograph of an arteriole illustrating endothelial cells (E) of the tunica intima (I), smooth muscle of the tunica media (M), and connective tissue of the tunica adventitia (Ad). V, venules; N, nerve bundle. Masson's stain. × 344.

FIGURE 11-21
Photomicrograph of a venule illustrating endothelial cells (E) of the extremely thin tunica intima (I), a few smooth muscle cells of the tunica media (M), and connective tissue of the tunica adventitia (Ad). Masson's stain. × 344.

FIGURE 11-22
Photomicrograph depicting three arterioles and a capillary (arrow). × 869.

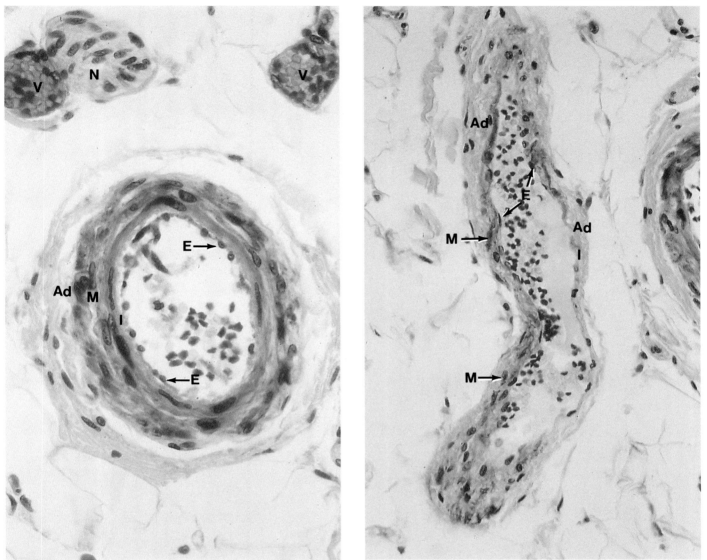

figure 11-20

figure 11-21

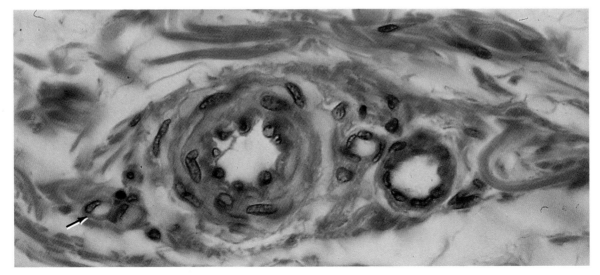

figure 11-22

FIGURE 11-23
Photomicrograph depicting capillaries (arrows) among profiles of cross-sectioned skeletal muscle (S). CT, connective tissue; F, fibroblasts; A, arteriole. × 560.

FIGURE 11-24
Photomicrograph of capillaries (arrows) among profiles of cross-sectioned cardiac muscle (C). × 1376.

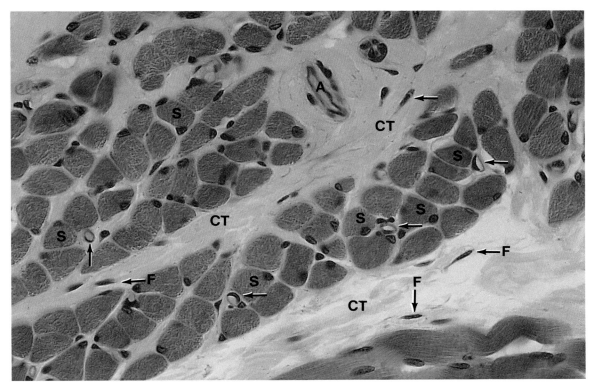

figure 11-23

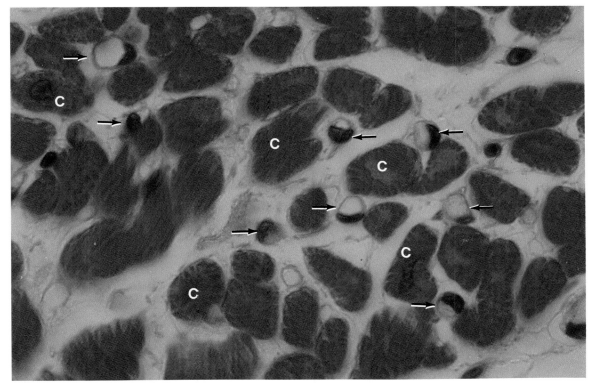

figure 11-24

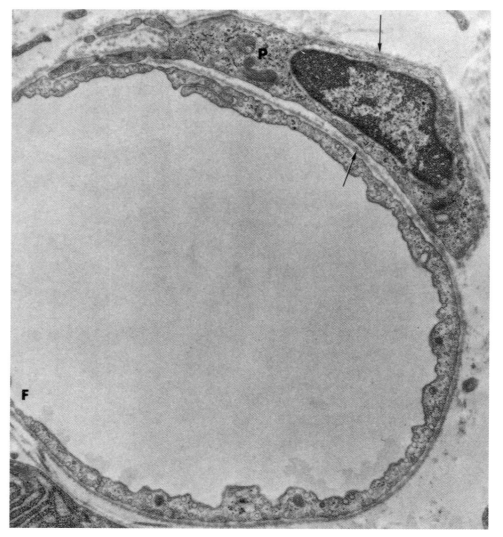

figure 11-25

FIGURE 11-25
Electron micrograph of a capillary from monkey pancreas showing fenestrations (F) and a pericyte (P). Note the basal lamina (arrows) on both sides of the pericyte. × 13,630. (Reprinted with permission from *Bailey's Textbook of Microscopic Anatomy*, 18th ed., by Douglas E. Kelly, Richard L. Wood, and Allen C. Enders. Williams & Wilkins, 1984.)

FIGURE 11-26
Electron micrograph of a continuous capillary in cross section showing tight junctions (TJ) and pinocytotic vesicles (P). Note the surrounding basal lamina (arrows) and erythrocyte (E) in the lumen of the vessel. Rat; × 15,698. (Courtesy of Ms. Susan Decker.)

FIGURE 11-27
Electron micrograph of a fenestrated capillary wall showing fenestrae with a thin diaphragm and the continuous underlying basal lamina. L, lumen of capillary; BL, basal lamina. × 67,500. (Reprinted with permission from *Bailey's Textbook of Microscopic Anatomy*, 18th ed., by Douglas E. Kelly, Richard L. Wood, and Allen C. Enders. Williams & Wilkins, 1984.)

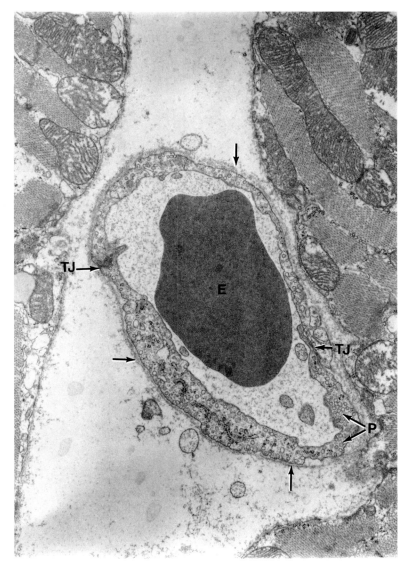

figure 11-26

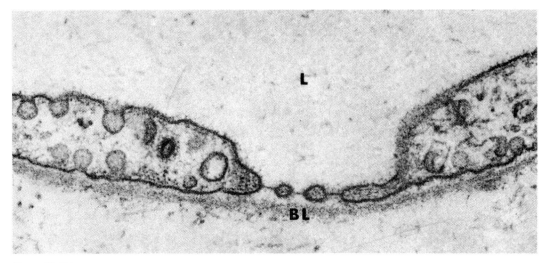

figure 11-27

FIGURE 11-28
Photomicrograph of a sinusoid (S) from the spleen. Note the endothelial cells (arrows) lining the lumen of the vessel. Plastic section. × 560.

FIGURE 11-29
Photomicrograph of a sinusoid from the liver. Note the endothelial cells (arrows) lining the sinusoidal lumen (S). × 560.

FIGURE 11-30
Photomicrograph of a lymphatic capillary (L). Note the endothelial cells (arrows) lining the capillary lumen. V, venules. × 344.

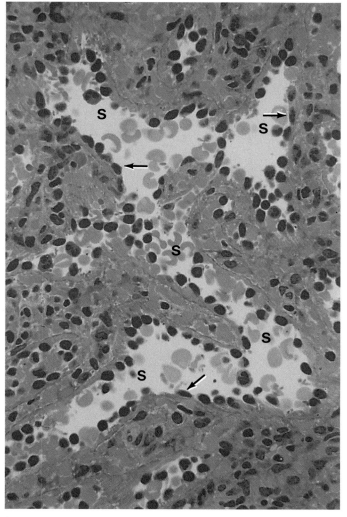

figure 11-28

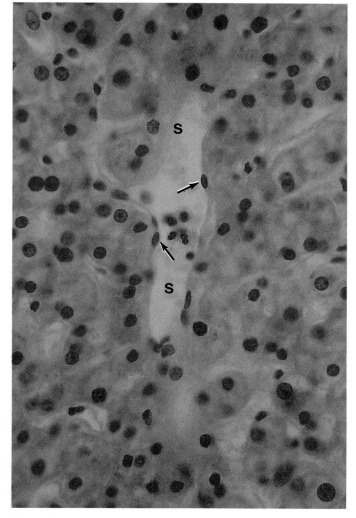

figure 11-29

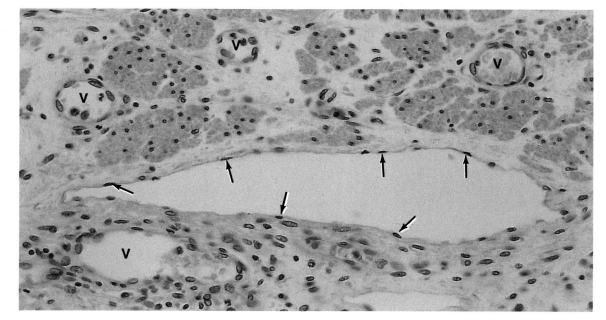

figure 11-30

FIGURE 12-1
Photomicrograph of the bell stage in tooth development. OEE, outer enamel epithelium; PD, predentin; A, ameloblast cell layer; O, odontoblast cell layer; DP, dental papilla; SR, stellate reticulum; DF, dental follicle; B, bone. Pig; × 56.

FIGURE 12-2
Photomicrograph of developing tooth illustrating enamel (E), dentin (D), ameloblast cell layer (A), odontoblast cell layer (O), and the dental papilla (DP). Pig; × 56.

FIGURE 12-3
Photomicrograph of a developing incisor (I) and molar (M) at the nineteenth day of gestation in the rat. DP, dental papilla; A, ameloblast cell layer; O, odontoblast cell layer; D, dentin; E, enamel; B, bone. Rat; × 56.

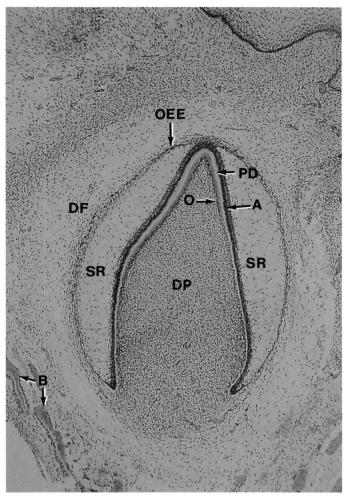

figure 12-1

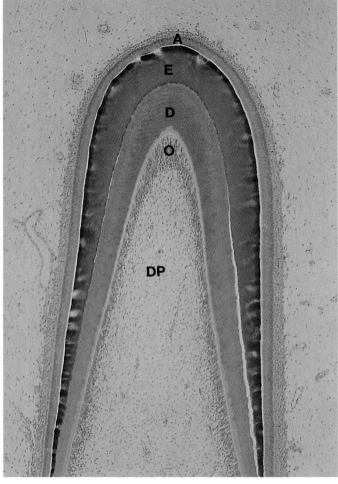

figure 12-2

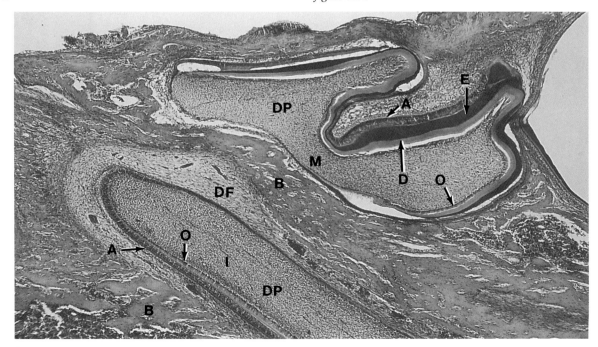

figure 12-3

FIGURE 12-4
Photomicrograph of part of the incisor shown in Figure 12-3. DP, dental papilla; O, odontoblast cell layer; PD, predentin; D, dentin; E, enamel; A, ameloblast cell layer; B, bone. Rat; × 140.

FIGURE 12-5
Higher-power photomicrograph of the area depicted in Figure 12-4. O, odontoblast cell layer; AS, artifactual space; PD, predentin; D, dentin; E, enamel; A, ameloblast cell layer; arrows, nuclei of cells of the stratum intermedium. Rat; × 560.

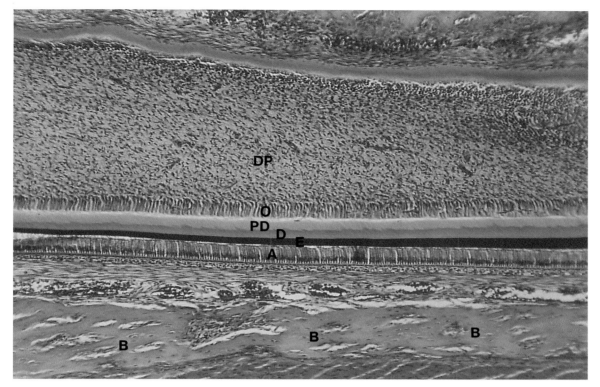

figure 12-4

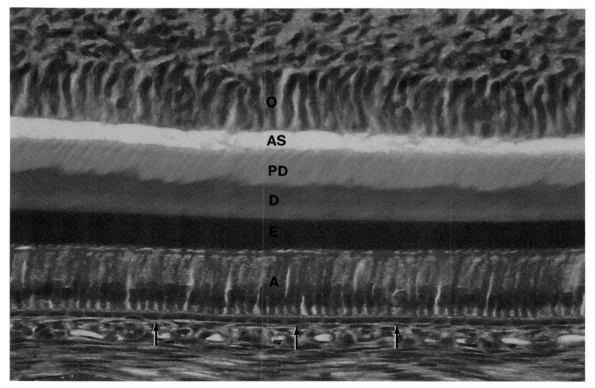

figure 12-5

FIGURE 12-6

Photomicrograph of a frontal section of an undecalcified unstained incisor tooth. C, crown; R, root; E, enamel; D, dentin; P, pulp. × 4.

FIGURE 12-7

Photomicrograph of a frontal section of an undecalcified unstained molar tooth. C, crown; R, root; E, enamel; D, dentin; P, pulp; arrow, cementum. × 4.

FIGURE 12-8

Higher magnification of part of the molar shown in Figure 12-7. E, enamel; arrow, dentinal–enamel junction; DT, dentinal tubules; P, pulp. × 12.

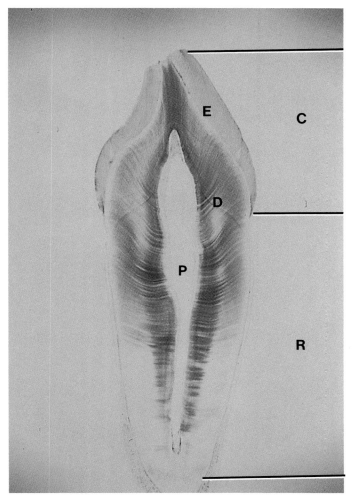

figure 12-6

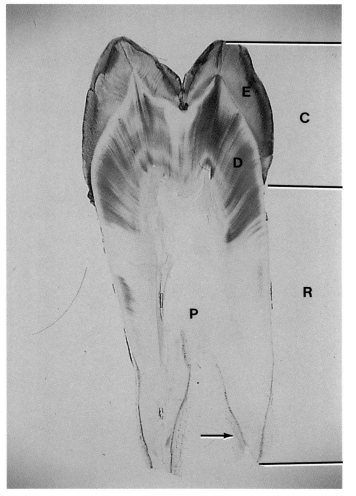

figure 12-7

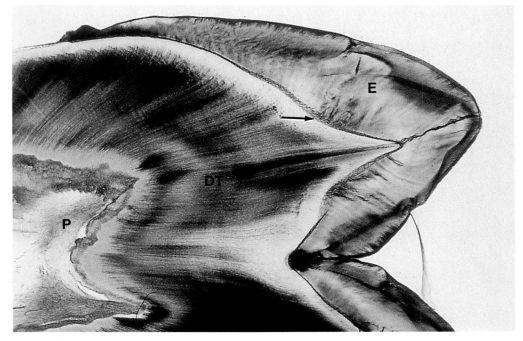

figure 12-8

FIGURE 12-9

Photomicrograph of part of the tongue illustrating filiform (Fi) and fungiform (F) papillae. Note the arrangement of its skeletal muscle (S). SS, stratified squamous epithelium; B, bone. Masson's stain. Embryonic mouse jaw; × 14.

FIGURE 12-10

Photomicrograph of part of the tongue showing filiform (Fi) and fungiform (F) papillae. SS, stratified squamous keratinized epithelium; CT, connective tissue. × 56.

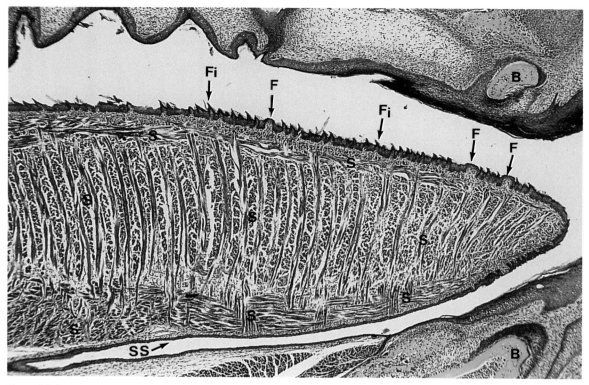

figure 12-9

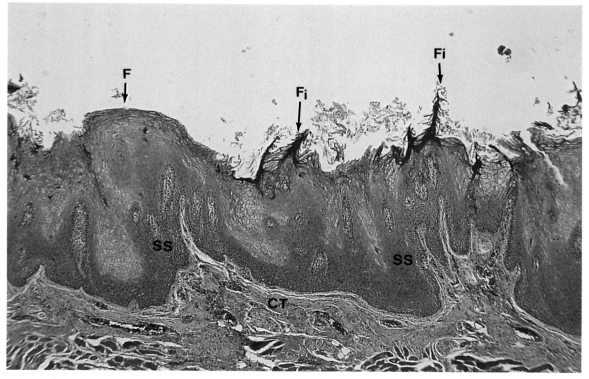

figure 12-10

FIGURE 12-11
Photomicrograph of part of a tongue illustrating filiform papillae. SS, stratified squamous keratinized epithelium; CT, connective tissue; S, skeletal muscle. Azure stain. Rat; × 140.

FIGURE 12-12
Photomicrograph of a circumvallate papilla showing stratified squamous epithelium (SS), taste buds (TB), connective tissue (CT), von Ebner's glands (GL), and skeletal muscle (S). For more details of taste buds, see Chapter 20, Figures 20-2–20-22. Monkey; × 56.

FIGURE 12-13
Photomicrograph of foliate papillae, which are not prominent in human tongue. SS, stratified squamous epithelium; CT, connective tissue; TB, taste buds; GL, von Ebner's glands; D, ducts of glands; S, skeletal muscle. Rabbit; × 140.

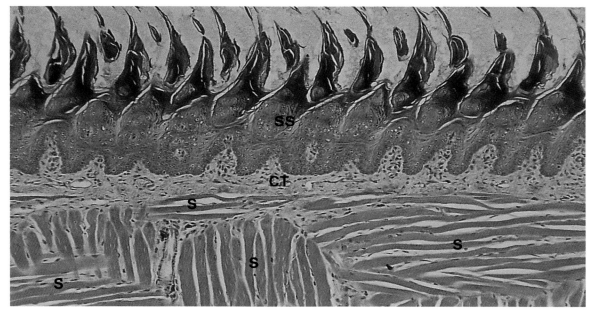

figure 12-11

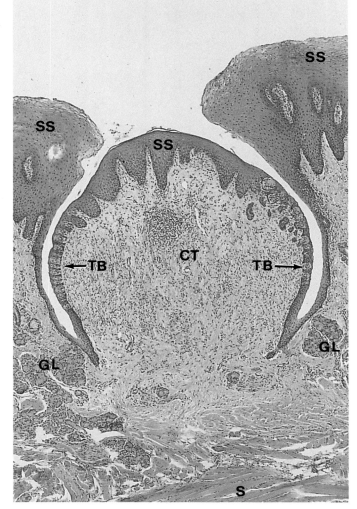

figure 12-12

figure 12-13

FIGURE 12-14

Scanning electron micrograph of the esophagus illustrating the four layers, mucosa (Mu), submucosa (Su), muscularis externa (ME), and adventia (serosa) (Ad), which is the basic architectural organization of the digestive tract from the esophagus through the large intestine. × 60. (Reprinted with permission from *Tissue and Organs: A Text-Atlas of Scanning Electron Microscopy,* by Richard G. Kessel and Randy H. Kardon. Copyright © 1979 W. H. Freeman & Company.)

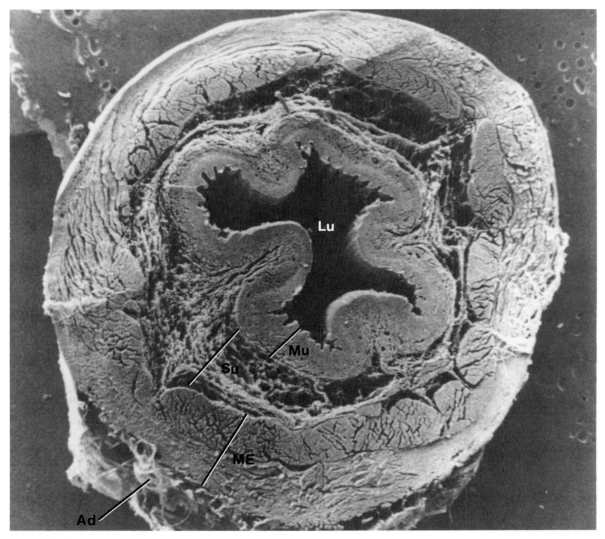

figure 12-14

FIGURE 12-15
Photomicrograph of a transverse section of the esophagus illustrating its four layers, mucosa (M), submucosa (SM), muscularis externa (ME), and adventitia (A). SS, stratified squamous epithelium of the mucosa. × 56.

FIGURE 12-16
Photomicrograph of a longitudinal section of the mucosa of the esophagus. SS, stratified squamous epithelium; LP, lamina propria; MM, muscularis mucosae. Also seen are the submucosal or esophageal glands proper (GL) and their ducts (D). × 140.

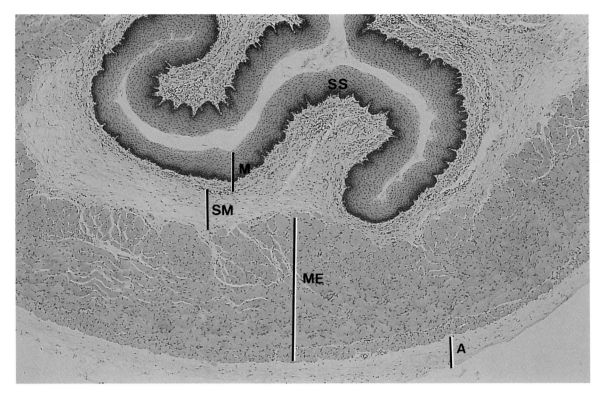

figure 12-15

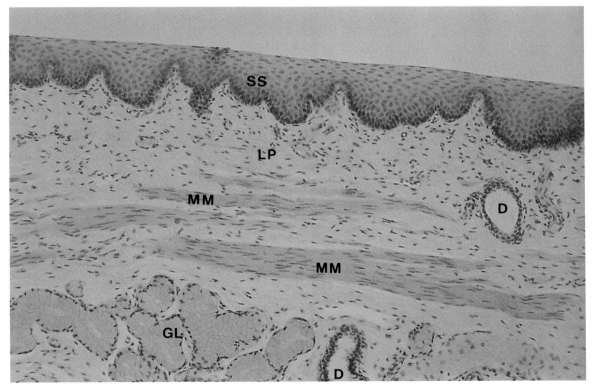

figure 12-16

FIGURE 12-17
Photomicrograph of the junction of the esophagus (E) with the stomach. Seen are the cardiac (C) and fundic (F) portions of the stomach, lamina propriae (LP), muscularis mucosae (MM), cardiac glands (arrows), esophageal glands proper (EG), submucosal connective tissue (CT), muscularis externa of the esophagus (MEE), and muscularis externa of the stomach (MES). Dog; × 14.

FIGURE 12-18
Photomicrograph of the junction of the esophagus (E) with cardiac stomach (C) showing gastric pits (GP), cardiac glands (CG), esophageal cardiac glands (ECG), muscularis mucosae (arrows), and submucosa (SM). Dog; × 56.

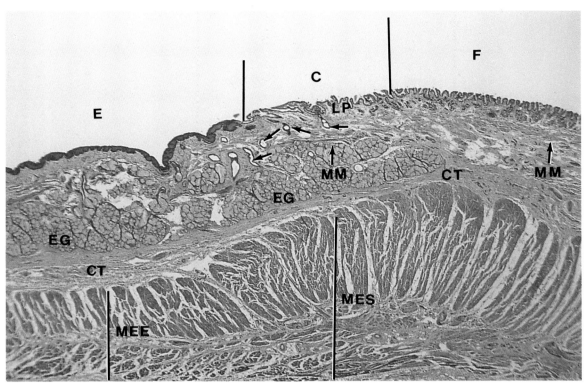

figure 12-17

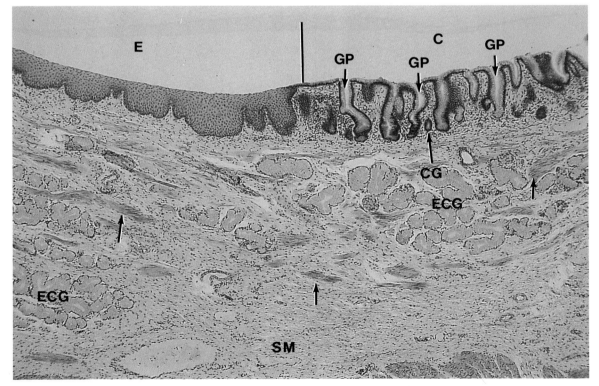

figure 12-18

FIGURE 12-19
Photomicrograph of the transition of the esophagus to the cardiac part of the stomach showing stratified squamous epithelium of the esophagus (SS), gastric pits (P), cardiac glands (CG), esophageal cardiac glands (ECG), muscularis mucosae (arrows), submucosa (SM), and muscularis externa (ME) of the stomach. Dog; × 56.

FIGURE 12-20
Higher-power photomicrograph of part of the cardiac stomach shown in Figure 12-19. Note the mucous surface epithelial cells (arrows), gastric pits (P), and cardiac glands (CG) in the lamina propria (LP). Dog; × 344.

FIGURE 12-21
Low-power photomicrograph illustrating the transition of the cardiac (C) part of the stomach to the fundic (F) part of the stomach. CG, cardiac glands; FG, fundic glands; arrows, muscularis mucosae; SM, submucosa; P, gastric pits. Dog; × 56.

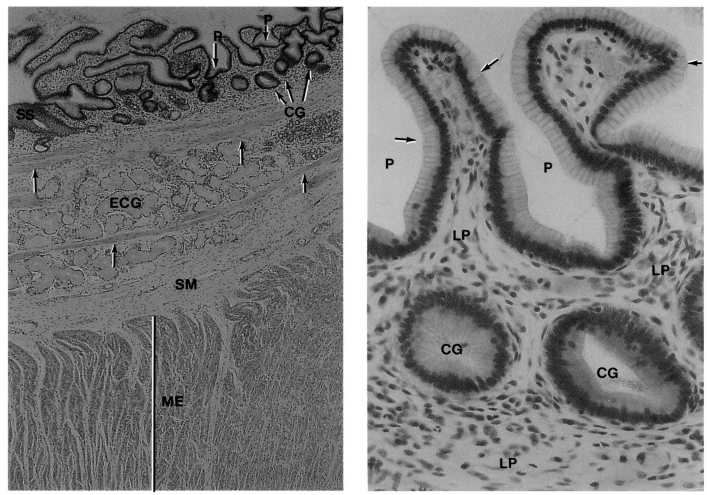

figure 12-19

figure 12-20

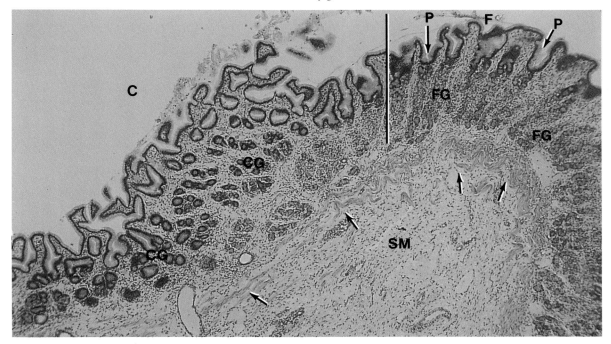

figure 12-21

FIGURE 12-22
Photomicrograph illustrating rugae of part of an undistended portion of fundic stomach. M, mucosa; arrows, muscularis mucosae; SM, submucosa; ME, muscularis externa; S, serosa; V, blood vessels. Dog; × 12.

FIGURE 12-23
Photomicrograph of part of a fundic gland showing mucus-secreting surface epithelial cells (M), gastric pit (P), mucous neck cells (MN), parietal cells (arrows), and chief cells (C). Dog; × 299.

FIGURE 12-24
Photomicrograph of part of a fundic gland showing chief (arrows) and parietal (P) cells. Dog; × 299.

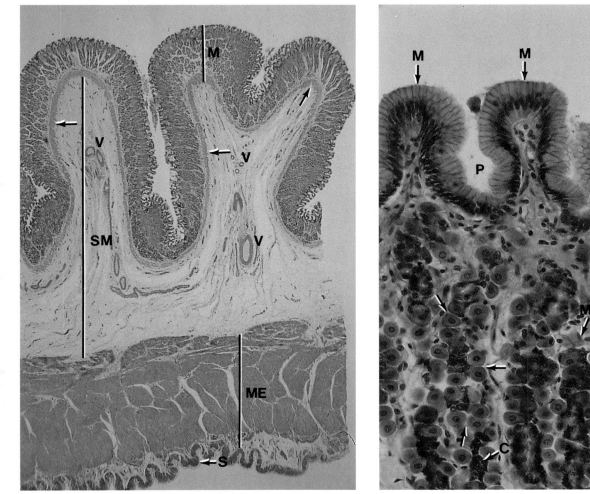

figure 12-22

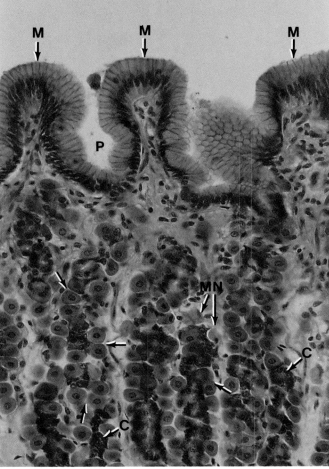

figure 12-23

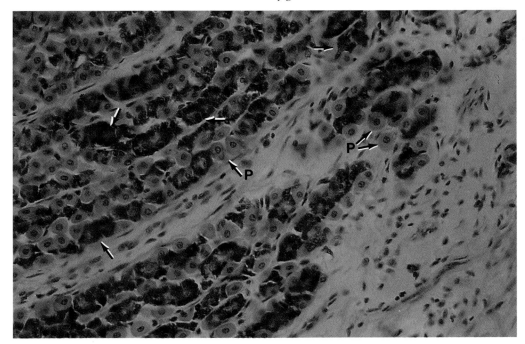

figure 12-24

FIGURE 12-25
Photomicrograph of the pyloric portion of the stomach showing the mucosa (M), sub-mucosa (SM), and muscularis externa (ME). Dog; × 56.

FIGURE 12-26
Higher-power photomicrograph of part of the pyloric stomach shown in Figure 12-25. GL, pyloric glands; P, pits; MM, muscularis mucosae. Dog; × 140.

FIGURE 12-27
Photomicrograph illustrating the junction (unlabeled arrow) of the pylorus with the duodenum, the initial segment of the small intestine. MEP, muscularis externa of the pylorus; PS, pyloric sphincter; B, Brunner's glands of the duodenum; V, villi of the duodenum; MED, muscularis externa of the duodenum. Dog; × 14.

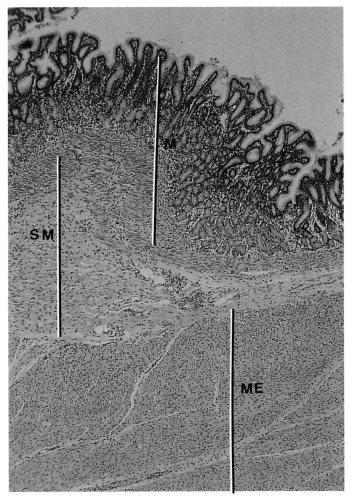

figure 12-25

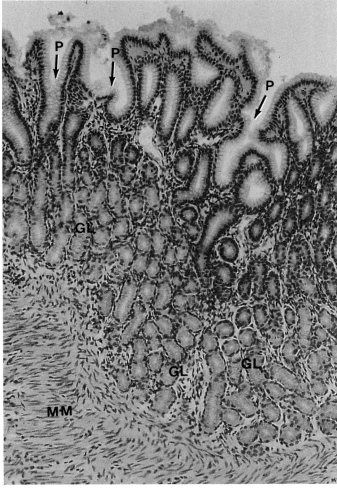

figure 12-26

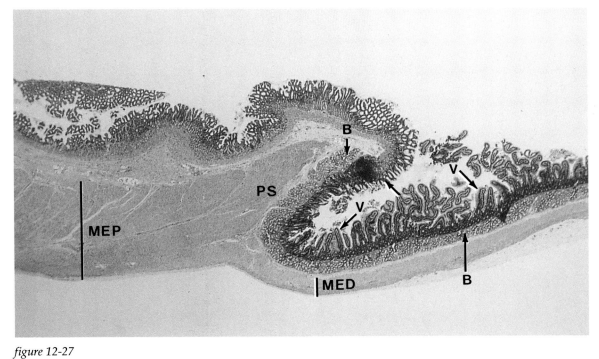

figure 12-27

FIGURE 12-28
Photomicrograph of the duodenum showing villi (V), Brunner's glands (B), plicae circulares (valves of Kerckring) (P), submucosa (S), muscularis external (ME), and mesentery (M). Pa, pancreas. Dog; × 14.

FIGURE 12-29
Photomicrograph of the jejunum illustrating villi (V), the muscularis externa (ME), and mesentery (M). Dog; × 14.

FIGURE 12-30
Photomicrograph of the ileum showing plicae circulares (valves of Kerckring) (P), villi (V), submucosa (S), muscularis externa (ME), Peyer's patches (arrows), and mesentery (M). Dog; × 14.

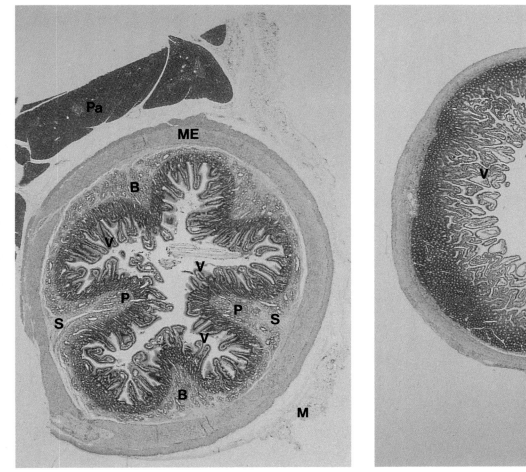

figure 12-28

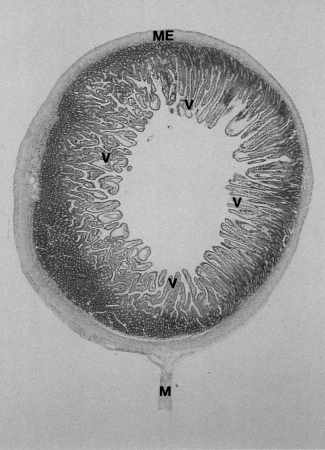

figure 12-29

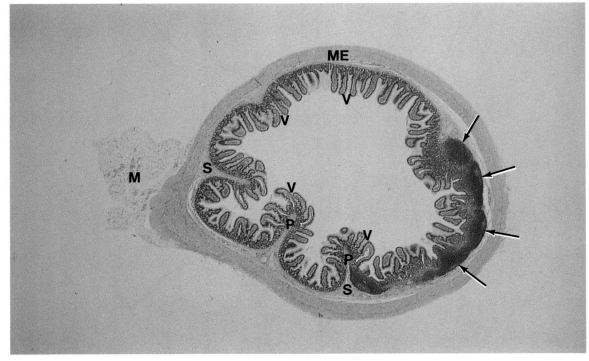

figure 12-30

FIGURE 12-31
Photomicrograph of the duodenum. Note Brunner's glands (B) in the submucosa (s). Also seen are villi (V), muscularis externa (ME), and crypts of Lieberkühn (arrows). Dog; ×49.

FIGURE 12-32
Photomicrograph of the jejunum. Note the finger-like shape of the villi (V). Also seen are the crypts of Lieberkühn (arrows), submucosa (s), and muscularis externa (ME). Dog; ×49.

FIGURE 12-33
Photomicrograph of the ileum. Note Peyer's patches (L), some of which have pale staining germinal centers. Also seen are villi (V), crypts of Lieberkühn (arrows), submucosa (s), and muscularis externa (ME). Dog; ×49.

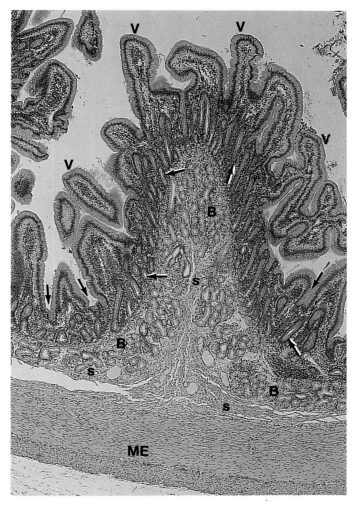

figure 12-31

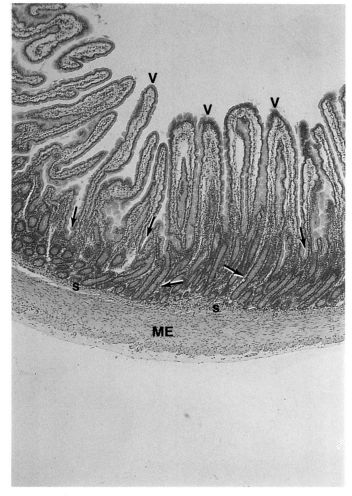

figure 12-32

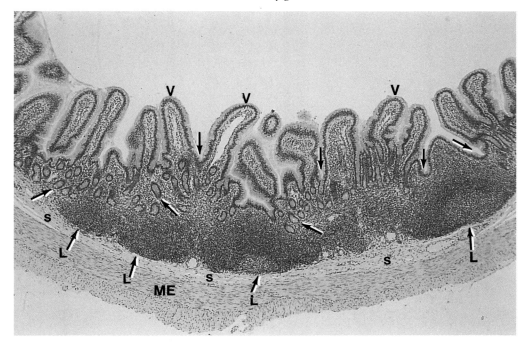

figure 12-33

FIGURE 12-34
Photomicrograph of the mucosa of the ileum. Note the goblet (G) and columnar absorbing (A) cells of the epithelium. Also seen are the lamina propria (LP), muscularis mucosae (MM), and crypts of Lieberkühn (arrows). × 140.

FIGURE 12-35
Photomicrograph of the base of two crypts of Lieberkühn of the ileum. Note the Paneth cells (P), goblet cells (G), lamina propria (LP), and blood vessel (V). × 560.

FIGURE 12-36
Cross section of an intestinal villus. Note the columnar absorbing (A) and goblet (G) cells of the epithelium. LP, lamina propria; V, blood vessels. × 344.

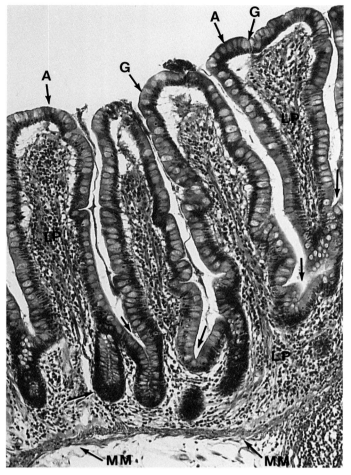

figure 12-34

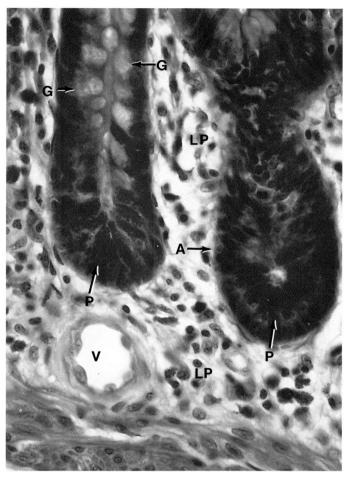

figure 12-35

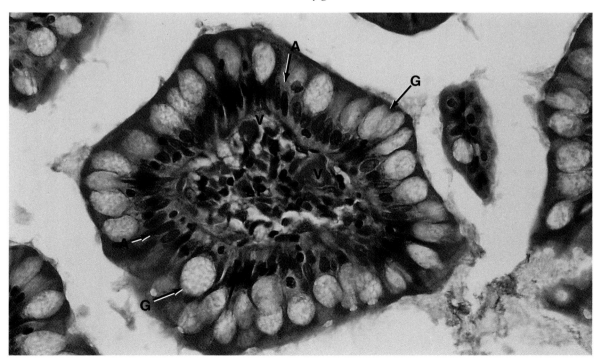

figure 12-36

FIGURE 12-37
Photomicrograph of a plica circularis (valve of Kerckring), a permanent fold of the mucosa (bar) and submucosa (S) of the small intestine. Also seen are villi (V), central lacteals (arrows), and muscularis externa (ME). Dog; × 56.

FIGURE 12-38
Photomicrograph of the tip of an intestinal villus. C, central lacteal; bar, lamina propria. Note the brush or striated border (arrows), lymphocyte (L) infiltration, and goblet cells (g) in the epithelium (E). Dog; × 344.

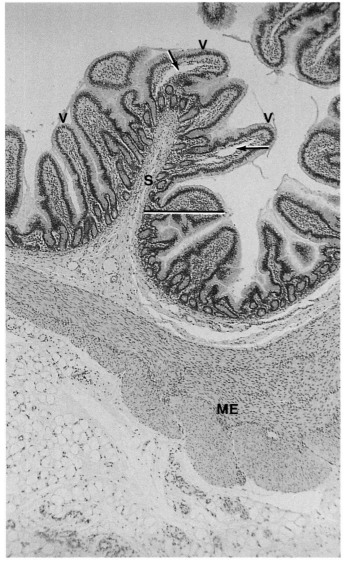

figure 12-37

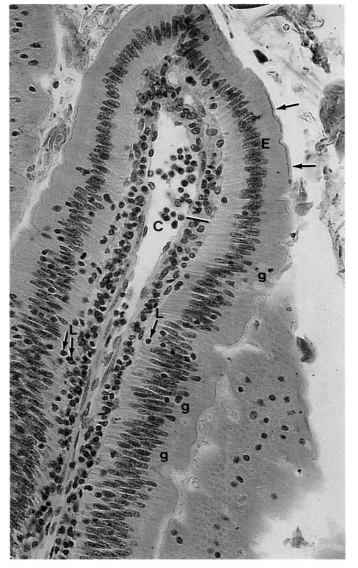

figure 12-38

FIGURE 12-39
Photomicrograph illustrating the submucosal (Meissner's) nerve plexus (arrows) between the submucosa (S) and inner circular (IC) layer of smooth muscle of the small intestine. OL, outer longitudinal smooth muscle; LN, lymph nodule. Dog; × 140.

FIGURE 12-40
Photomicrograph of the myenteric (Auerbach's) nerve plexus (arrows) between the inner circular (IC) and outer longitudinal (OL) layers of smooth muscle of the small intestine. S, submucosa. Dog; × 140.

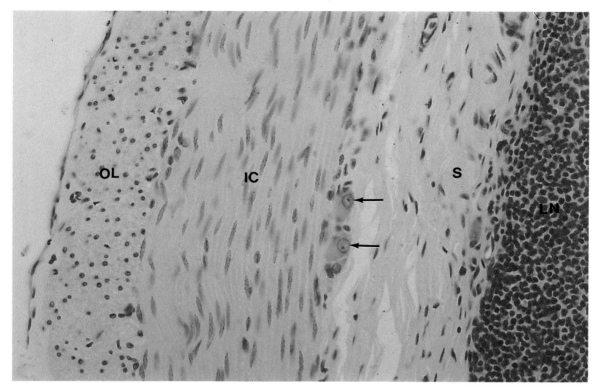

figure 12-39

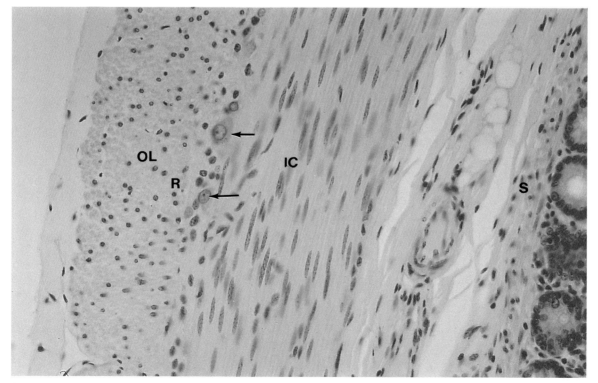

figure 12-40

FIGURE 12-41
Photomicrograph of the large intestine showing the mucosa (M), submucosa (S), and muscularis externa (ME). × 14.

FIGURE 12-42
Photomicrograph showing the mucosa (M) and submucosa (S) of the large intestine. The mucosal glands contain abundant goblet cells (arrows). MM, muscularis mucosae. × 56.

FIGURE 12-43
Transverse section of large intestine mucosal glands. Note the abundance of goblet cells (G). A, columnar absorbing cells; LP, lamina propria. × 344.

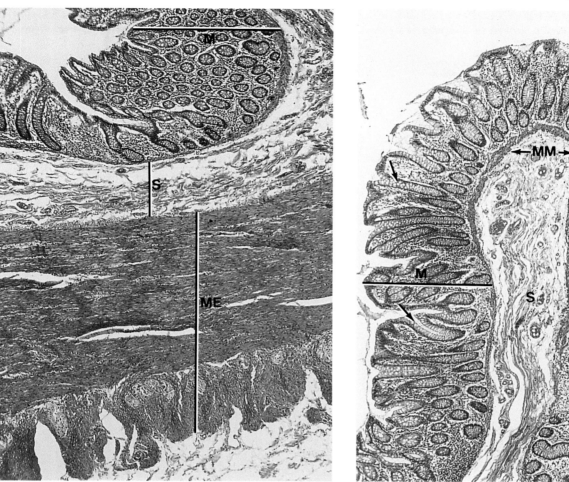

figure 12-41

figure 12-42

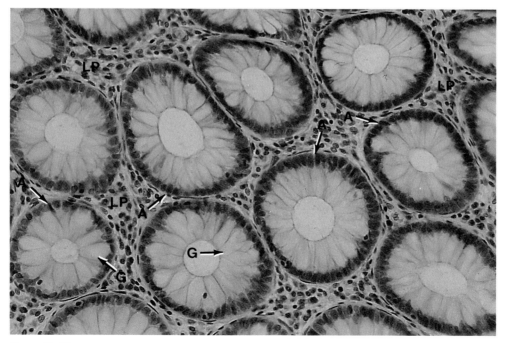

figure 12-43

FIGURE 13-1

Photomicrograph of part of the human liver. Although the micrograph is suggestive of a lobulated pattern of the parenchyma (P), the paucity of connective tissue in the human liver does not make for well-defined lobular boundaries. Evident are central veins (C) and portal triads (T). × 14.

FIGURE 13-2

Photomicrograph of pig liver illustrating lobules (L) whose boundaries are distinctly delimited by interlobular connective tissue (CT). C, central vein. × 56.

FIGURE 13-3

Photomicrograph of a liver lobule illustrating its roughly hexagonal shape, which is well delineated from adjacent lobules (L) by connective tissue (CT). Note the portal triads (T), which are better seen in Figures 13-4–13-7, and a central vein (C). Pig; × 140.

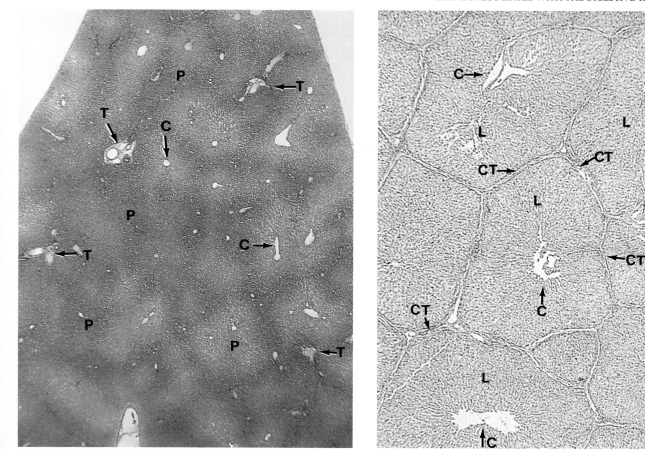

figure 13-1

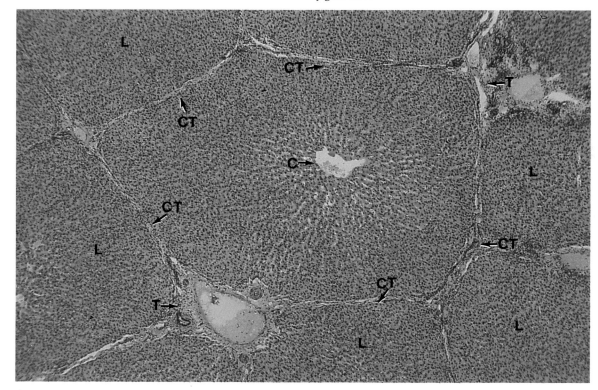

figure 13-2

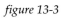

figure 13-3

FIGURE 13-4
Photomicrograph illustrating the components of a portal triad: bile ducts (D), a branch of the portal vein (V), and a branch of the hepatic artery (A). P, liver parenchyma; C, central vein. × 56.

FIGURE 13-5
Photomicrograph showing the plate-like or cordal arrangement of parenchymal liver cells (P). The space between cords of hepatocytes represents liver sinusoids. Note the bile duct (D), branch of the hepatic artery (A), and branch of the portal vein (V) of a portal triad. C, central vein. × 140.

FIGURE 13-6
High-power photomicrograph of a portal triad showing bile ducts (D), branch of the hepatic artery (A), and branch of the portal vein (V). Note the sinusoidal space (S) between hepatocytes. × 344.

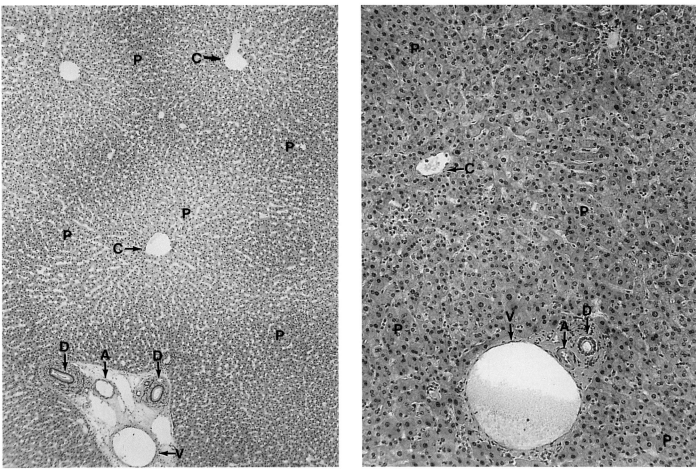

figure 13-4

figure 13-5

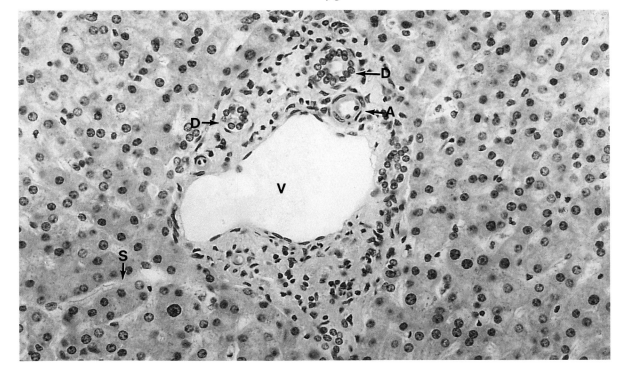

figure 13-6

FIGURE 13-7
Photomicrograph illustrating the direction of blood flow (arrow) from the branch of the portal vein (V) toward sinusoids (S) in the liver. D, bile duct; A, branch of the hepatic artery. × 344.

FIGURE 13-8
Photomicrograph illustrating the direction of blood flow (arrows) from sinusoids (S) to the central vein (V) of the liver. × 140.

FIGURE 13-9
High-power photomicrograph showing a sinusoid (arrow) emptying into the central vein (V) of the liver. × 344.

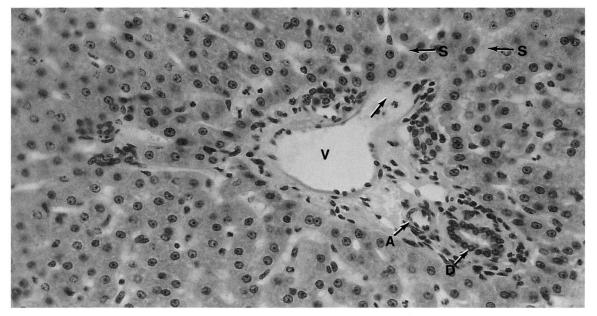

figure 13-7

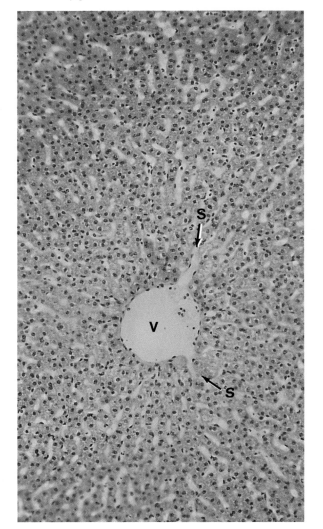

figure 13-8

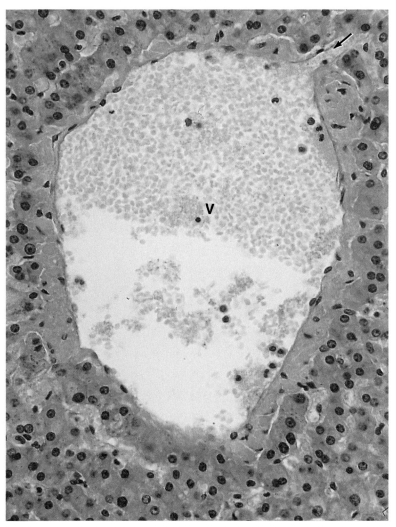

figure 13-9

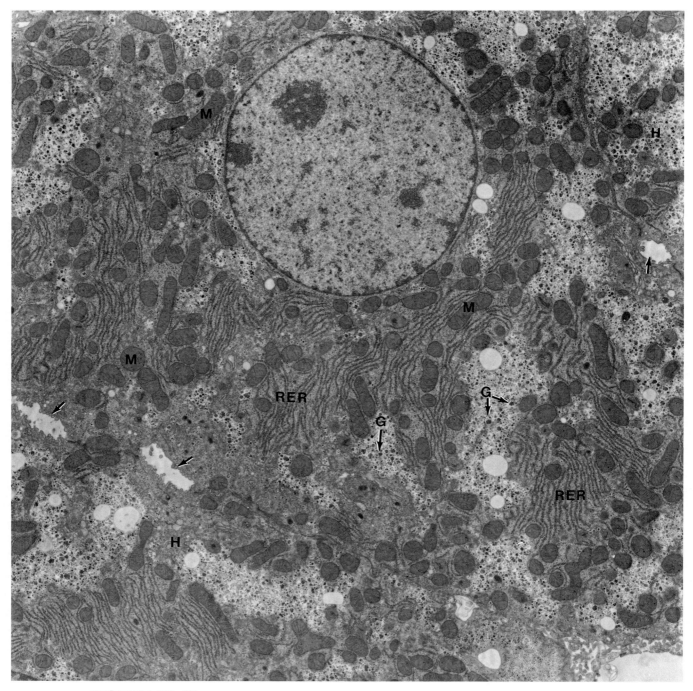

FIGURE 13-10
Electron micrograph of a hepatocyte and part of two adjoining hepatocytes (H). Note the bile canaliculi (arrows) along intercellular borders. M, mitochondria; RER, rough endoplasmic reticulum; G, glycogen. Rat; × 5820. (Courtesy of Dr. Richard L. Wood.)

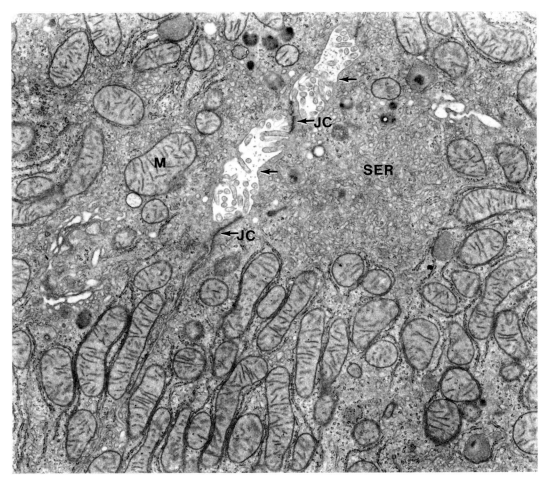

FIGURE 13-11
Electron micrograph illustrating bile canaliculi with prominent microvilli (arrows). Note the junctional complexes (JC). M, mitochondria; SER, smooth endoplasmic reticulum. Rat; × 12,250. (Courtesy of Dr. Richard L. Wood.)

FIGURE 13-12
Photomicrograph of part of the liver from a rat injected with the vital dye trypan blue. Note the phagocytic (Kupffer) cells (arrows), which have ingested the blue dye. Note also the anastomosing cords of hepatocytes (H) that delimit the liver sinusoidal space (S). Rat; × 344.

FIGURE 13-13
Photomicrograph of a Kupffer cell (arrow) from a rat that was injected with india ink. The phagocytosed ink particles almost obscure the nucleus of the cell. Note the surrounding hepatocytes (H), one of which is binucleate (BH). S, sinusoidal space. Rat; × 1376.

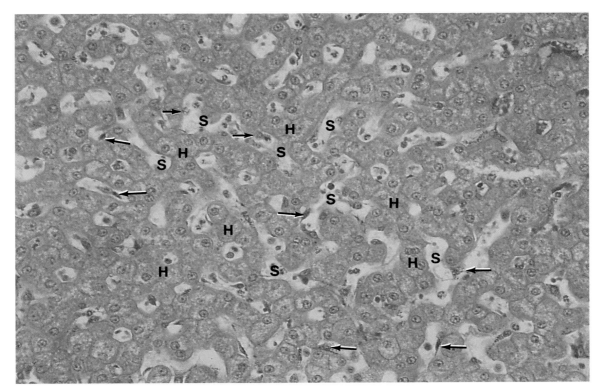

figure 13-12

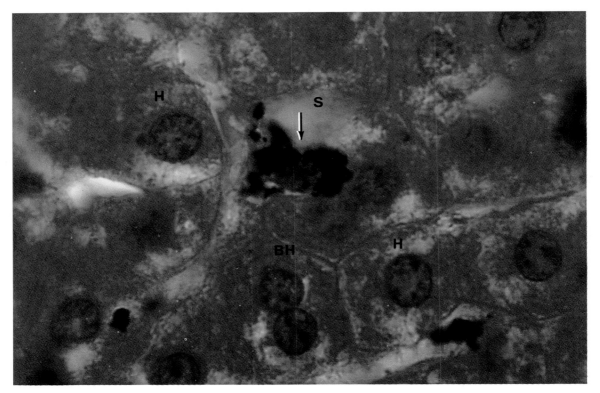

figure 13-13

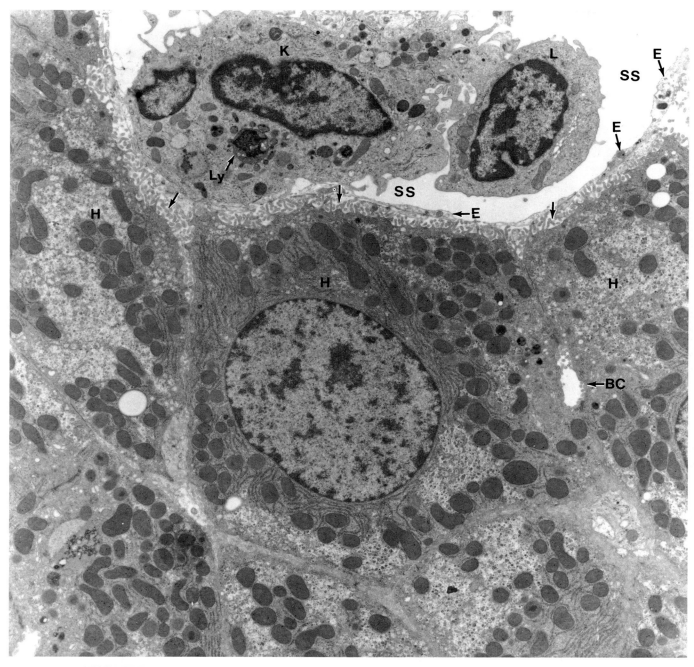

FIGURE 13-14

Electron micrograph illustrating the relationship between a sinusoid, the space of Disse, and hepatocytes in the liver. Note how the microvilli of the hepatocytes (H) project into the space of Disse (arrows), which separates the hepatocytes from the cell processes (E) of endothelial cells that line the sinusoidal space (SS). Note also the Kupffer cell (K) with a lysosome (Ly) and a lymphocyte (L) in the sinusoid. BC, bile canaliculus. Mouse; × 5640. (Courtesy of Dr. Richard L. Wood.)

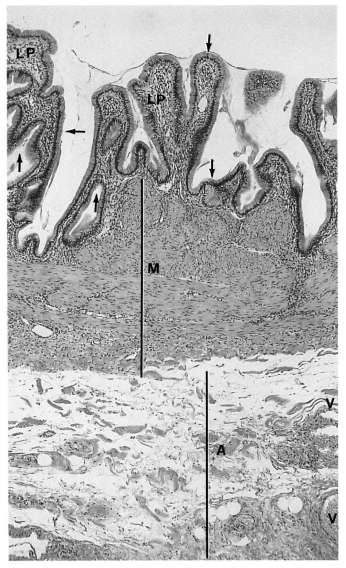

figure 13-15

figure 13-16

FIGURE 13-15

Photomicrograph of the wall of the gallbladder. The folded mucosa is composed of a simple columnar epithelium (arrows) and a lamina propria (LP). Directly beneath the lamina propria is the muscularis (M). Beneath the muscularis is the adventitia (A). Note the blood vessels (V) in the adventitia. × 56.

FIGURE 13-16

Higher-power photomicrograph of the epithelium (arrows), lamina propria (LP), and part of the muscularis (M) of the gallbladder depicted in Figure 13-15. × 140.

FIGURE 13-17
Photomicrograph of the pancreas illustrating serous acini (A), which with their ducts (D) represent the exocrine portion of the gland, and islets of Langerhans (I), which are the endocrine components of the gland. V, blood vessels. × 56.

FIGURE 13-18
Photomicrograph illustrating serous acini (A), intralobular ducts (D), and an islet of Langerhans in the pancreas. V, blood vessels. × 140.

FIGURE 13-19
Photomicrograph showing three small intralobular ducts (D), serous acini (A), and part of an islet of Langerhans of the pancreas. F, fat cell. × 344.

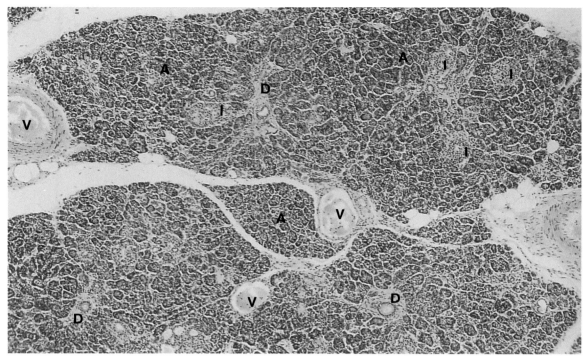

figure 13-17

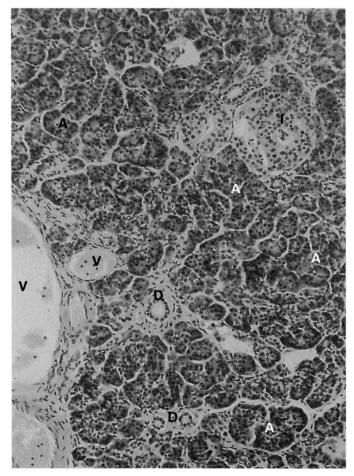

figure 13-18

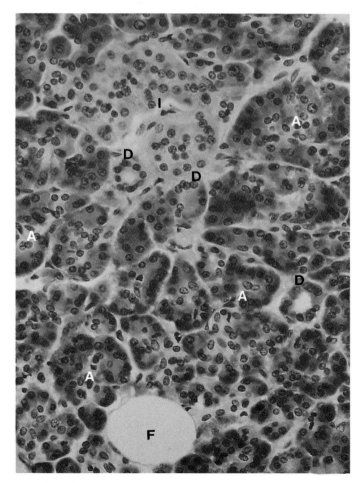

figure 13-19

FIGURE 13-20
Photomicrograph contrasting an intralobular duct (arrow) with an interlobular duct (D) in the pancreas. A, serous acini; I, islet of Langerhans; CT, connective tissue. × 140.

FIGURE 13-21
Photomicrograph illustrating centroacinar cells (arrows), serous acini (A), and fibroblasts (F) in the pancreas. × 344.

FIGURE 13-22
High-power photomicrograph showing centroacinar cells (arrows), the cells of serous acini (A), and fibroblasts (F) in the pancreas. × 1376.

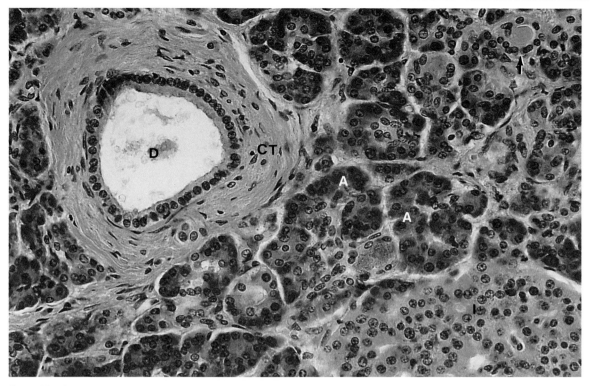

figure 13-20

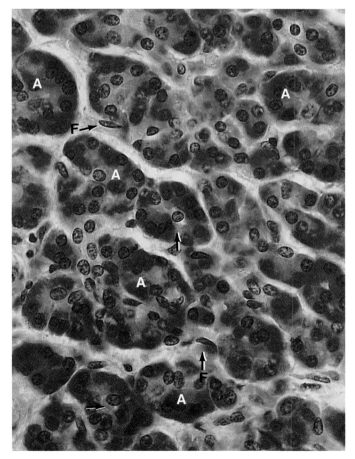

figure 13-21

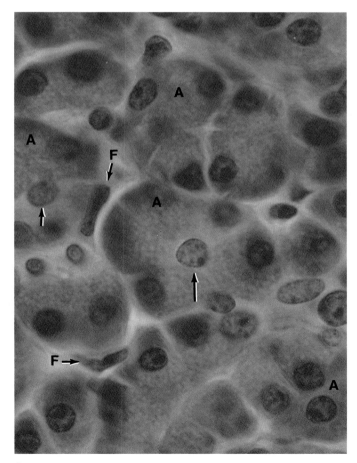

figure 13-22

FIGURE 13-23
Photomicrograph depicting serous acini (A), intralobular ducts (ID), and an interlobular duct (D) of the parotid. CT, connective tissue; V, blood vessel. × 56.

FIGURE 13-24
Photomicrograph of a part of the parotid illustrating serous acini (A), intralobular ducts (ID), interlobular ducts (D), blood vessels (V), and connective tissue (CT). × 140.

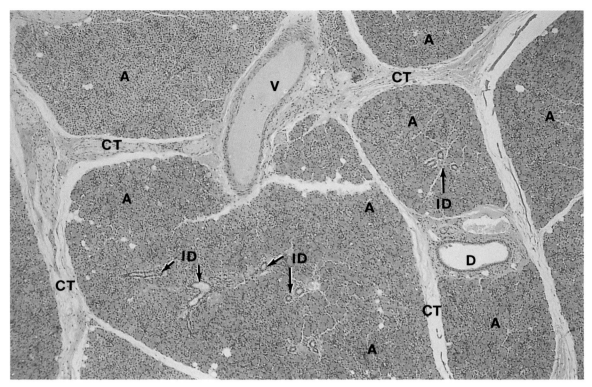

figure 13-23

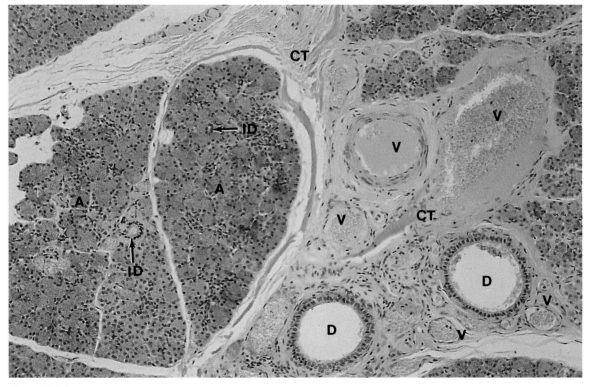

figure 13-24

FIGURE 13-25
Photomicrograph of an intercalated duct (arrow) and serous acini (A) of the parotid.
× 344.

FIGURE 13-26
Photomicrograph of striated ducts (arrows) and serous acini (A) in the parotid. CT, connective tissue. × 560.

FIGURE 13-27
Photomicrograph of an interlobular duct (D) in the parotid. Note the nerve bundles (N), blood vessels (V), connective tissue (CT), and intralobular ducts (ID). A, serous acini. × 140.

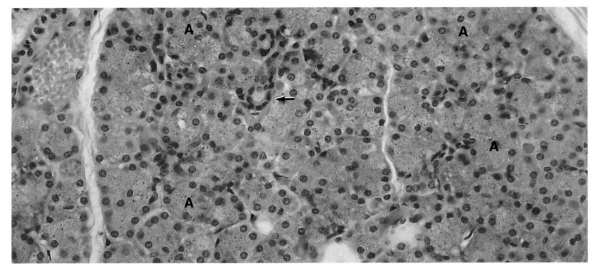

figure 13-25

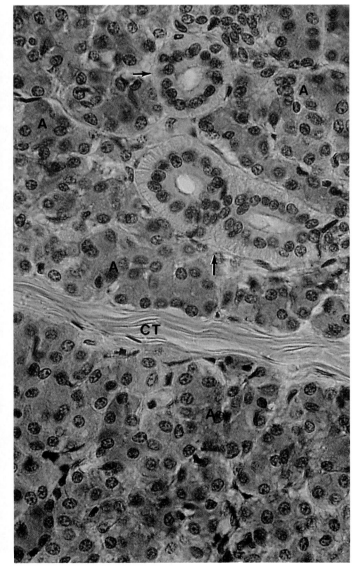

figure 13-26

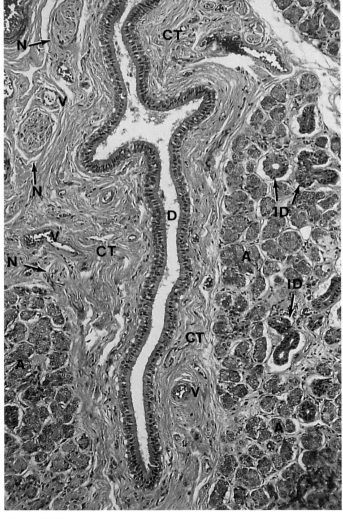

figure 13-27

FIGURE 13-28
Photomicrograph illustrating serous acini (A) and mixed serous and mucous acini (Mi) of the submandibular (submaxillary) gland. Note the numerous profiles of intralobular ducts (arrows) and an interlobular duct (D). × 56.

FIGURE 13-29
Higher-power photomicrograph of a portion of Figure 13-28 illustrating the serous cells (S) of serous demilunes which cap the mucous acini (M) of the submandibular gland. Note the intralobular ducts (ID). × 344.

FIGURE 13-30
Plastic section of the submandibular gland illustrating mucous acini (M), caping serous cells (S), serous acini (A), intralobular ducts (ID), and blood vessel (V). × 344.

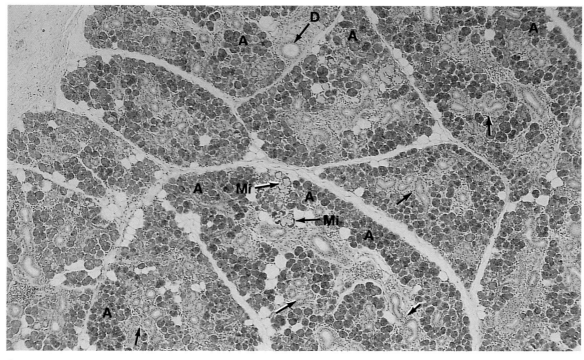

figure 13-28

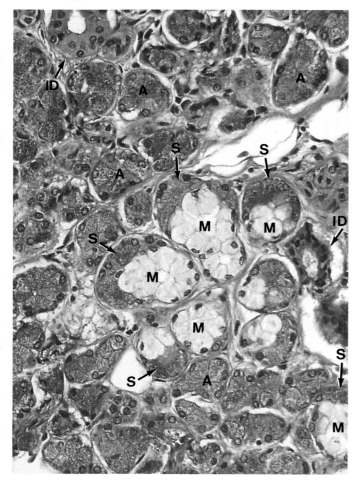

figure 13-29

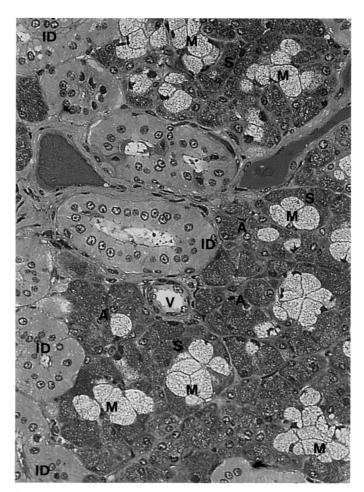

figure 13-30

FIGURE 13-31
Photomicrograph of part of the sublingual gland illustrating mucous acini (M), intralobular ducts (ID), and an interlobular duct (D) surrounded by skeletal muscle (SM). CT,
connective tissue. × 56.

FIGURE 13-32
Photomicrograph of the mucous acini (M) and intralobular ducts (ID) of the sublingual
gland. SM, skeletal muscle. × 140.

FIGURE 13-33
Photomicrograph of part of the sublingual gland showing mucous acini (M), some of
which are capped by serous demilunes (S). ID, intralobular duct; CT, connective tissue.
× 40.

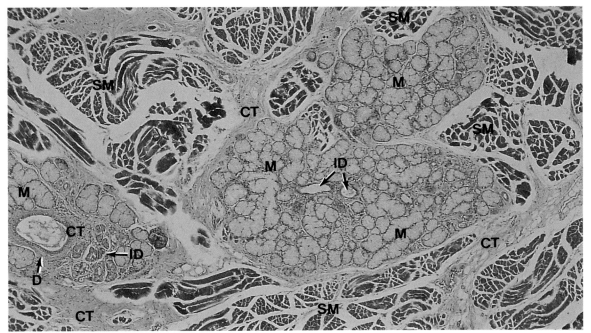

figure 13-31

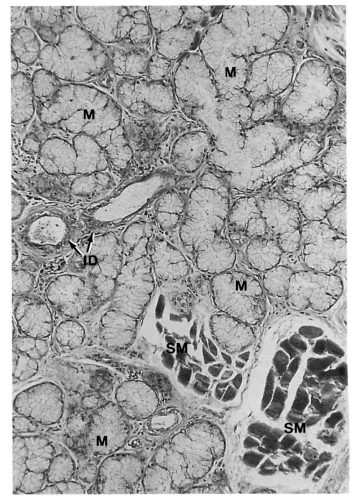

figure 13-32

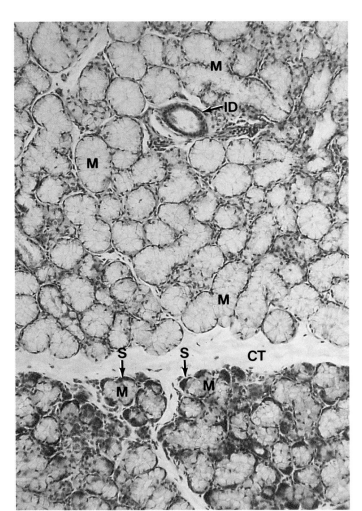

figure 13-33

FIGURE 14-1

Photomicrograph of a frontal section of the larynx illustrating the false vocal cords, the ventricular folds (VF), and the true vocal cords, the vocal folds (VoF). Also seen are ventricles (V), vocalis muscles (VM), mucoserous glands (GL), and a lymphatic nodule (LN). × 14.

FIGURE 14-2

Photomicrograph of a portion of the roof of the larynx showing seromucous glands (GL) and duct (D). Note the pseudostratified columnar epithelium (arrows) of this part of the larynx. Also seen are part of the epiglottis (E), connective tissue (CT), and blood vessels (v). × 56.

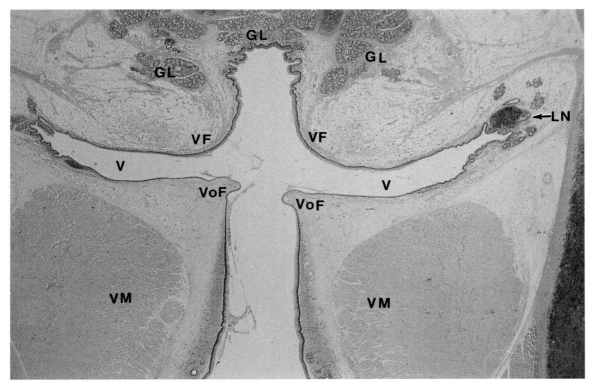

figure 14-1

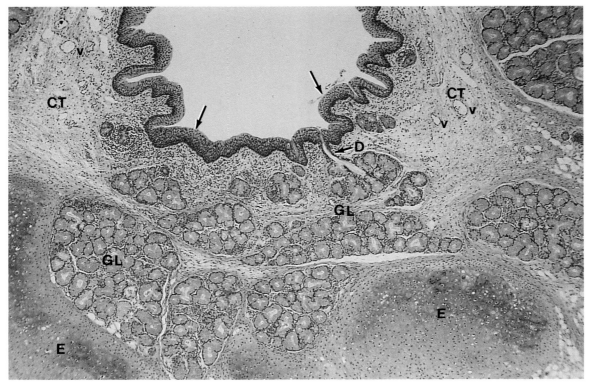

figure 14-2

FIGURE 14-3
Enlarged area of part of Figure 14-1 showing the transition (arrows) of pseudostratified columnar epithelium (PSC) in a laryngeal ventricle (V) to stratified squamous epithelium (SS). Also seen are connective tissue (CT), fat (F), and a lymphatic nodule (LN). × 56.

FIGURE 14-4
Photomicrograph of part of a laryngeal ventricle (V) illustrating pseudostratified columnar epithelium (arrows), glands (GL), a duct (D), subepithelial connective tissue (CT), fat (F), and blood vessels (Ve). × 140.

FIGURE 14-5
Photomicrograph of part of the nasal concha illustrating olfactory (O) and respiratory (R) mucosae. At the unlabeled arrow there is a transition of respiratory epithelium to olfactory epithelium. G, goblet cells; B, bone. For more details of respiratory and olfactory epithelia, see Chapter 20, Figures 20-12–20-14. × 140.

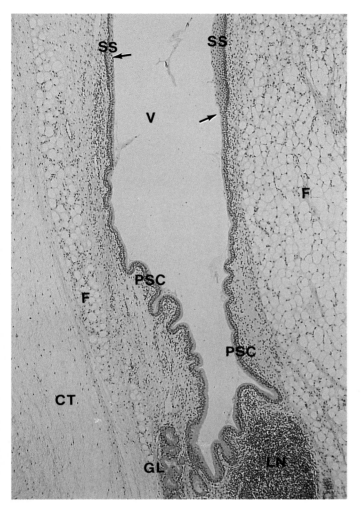

figure 14-3

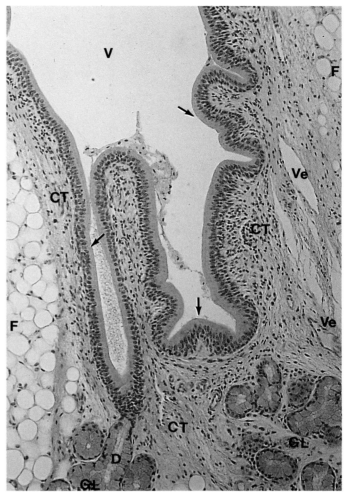

figure 14-4

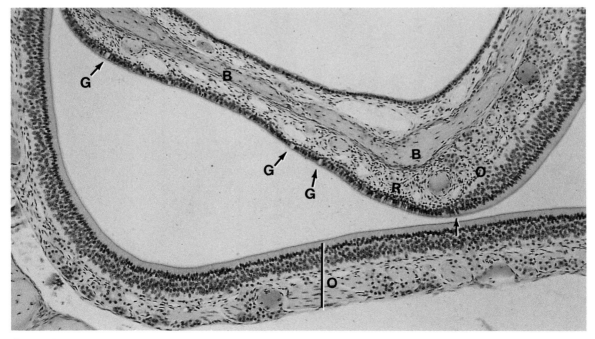

figure 14-5

FIGURE 14-6

Low-power photomicrograph of part of the trachea illustrating its relatively thin mucosal (M) and thick submucosal (SM) layers. Note the goblet cells (arrows) in the mucosal epithelium and the perichondrium (PC) of a part of a tracheal hyaline cartilage (HC) ring. Note also the numerous blood vessels (V) in the submucosa, which are not always observed in the trachea. F, fat. × 56.

FIGURE 14-7

Photomicrograph illustrating the mucous (M) and seromucous (SM) components of tracheal submucosal (S) glands. Note the duct (D) of a gland and lymphocyte aggregates (L) in the mucosal lamina propria (LP). E, epithelium. × 140.

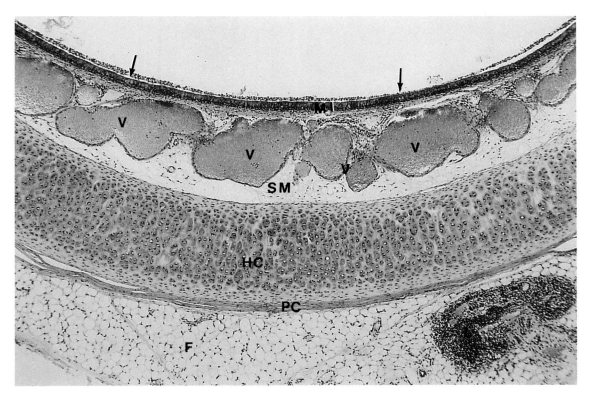

figure 14-6

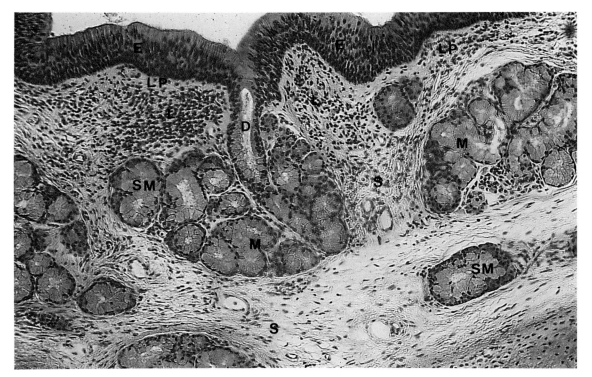

figure 14-7

FIGURE 14-8
Photomicrograph illustrating goblet cells (G), ciliated columnar cells (C), and basal cells (B) of the tracheal epithelium. Note the thick basement membrane (BM) and numerous blood vessels (V) in the lamina propria (LP) of the trachea. × 344.

FIGURE 14-9
Photomicrograph illustrating a brush cell (BC) cilia of columnar cells (C), and basal cells (B) in the epithelium of the trachea. LP, lamina propria. This part of the trachea lacks visible goblet cells. × 869.

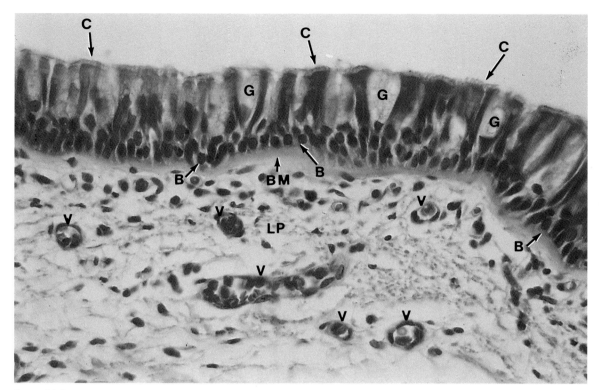

figure 14-8

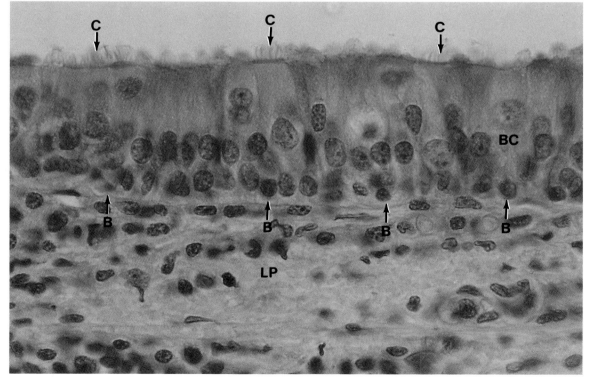

figure 14-9

FIGURE 14-10

Photomicrograph of a bronchus. Seen are epithelium (E), smooth muscle (SM), submucosal glands (GL), hyaline cartilage (C), and blood vessels (V). Note the surrounding lung tissue (LT). × 56.

FIGURE 14-11

Higher-power photomicrograph of part of the bronchus shown in Figure 14-10. Note the pseudostratified ciliated columnar epithelium (E), the smooth muscle (SM) bundles in the lamina propria (LP), and bars of hyaline cartilage (C). GL, submucosal glands; LT, lung tissue. × 140.

FIGURE 14-12

Photomicrograph of the bronchial respiratory epithelium. Note the goblet cells (G), which because of the thickness of the section appear heavily ciliated, ciliated columnar cells (arrows), and smooth muscle (SM) bundles in the underlying lamina propria (LP). GL, glands; C, hyaline cartilage. × 560.

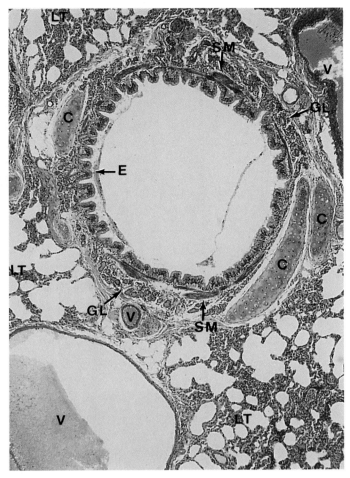

figure 14-10

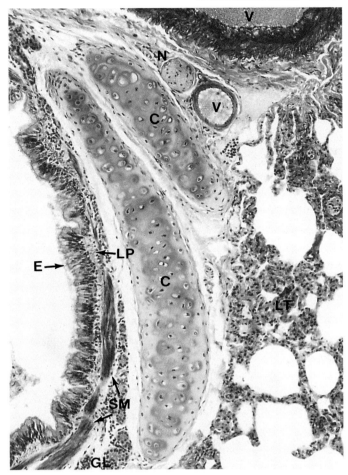

figure 14-11

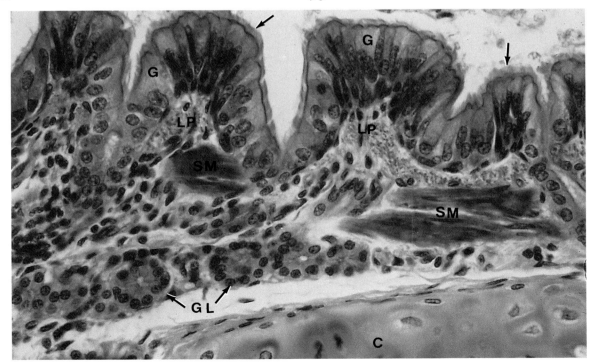

figure 14-12

FIGURE 14-13

Photomicrograph illustrating the characteristic folded epithelium (E) and prominent smooth muscle (arrows) of a bronchiole. Note the absence of hyaline cartilage and submucosal glands in the bronchiole wall. LP, lamina propria; CT, connective tissue; LT, lung tissue. × 140.

FIGURE 14-14

Photomicrograph of a small bronchiole. The epithelium (E) is cuboidal in a structure of this size. Note the diminished layers of smooth muscle cells (arrows). × 344.

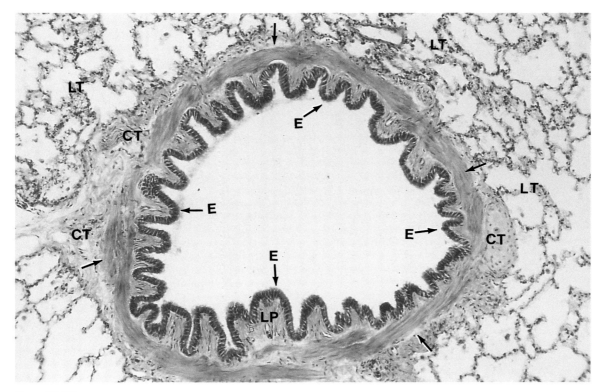

figure 14-13

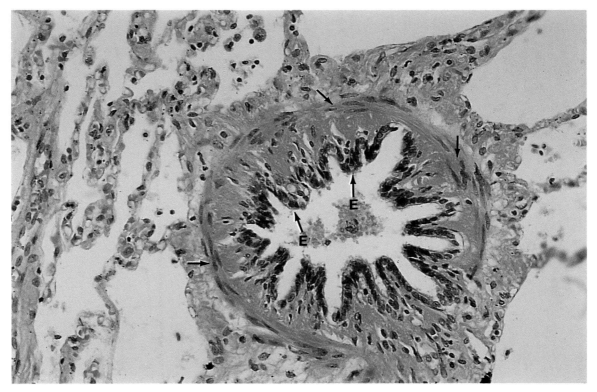

figure 14-14

FIGURE 14-15

Photomicrograph illustrating a bronchiole (B) and terminal bronchiole (TB) leading into a respiratory bronchiole (RB), which in turn leads into an alveolar duct (AD). E, bronchiolar epithelium; arrows, smooth muscle. × 12.

FIGURE 14-16

Higher-power photomicrograph of part of Figure 14-15 showing part of a terminal bronchiole (TB), a respiratory bronchiole (RB), and an alveolar duct (AD). Also seen are smooth muscle (arrows), alveoli (A), and blood vessels (V). × 122.

FIGURE 14-17

Photomicrograph of a respiratory bronchiole (RB). Note the cuboidal epithelium (C) and smooth muscle (arrows) of the respiratory bronchiolar wall. V, blood vessels. × 122.

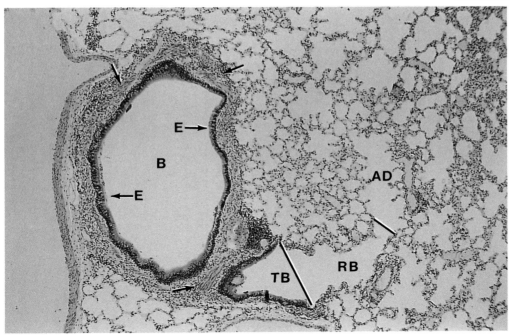

figure 14-15

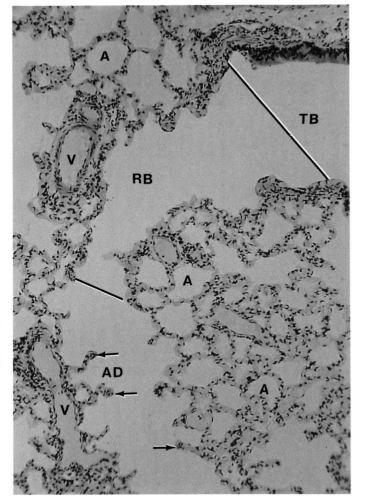

figure 14-16

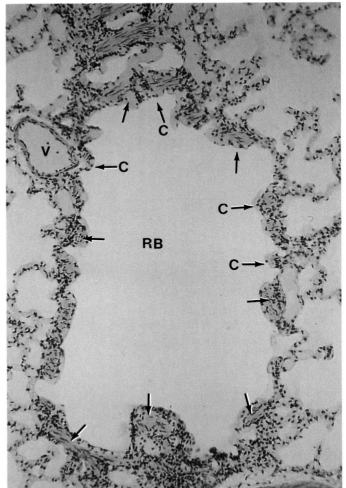

figure 14-17

FIGURE 14-18
Photomicrograph showing a respiratory bronchiole (RB) branching into alveolar ducts (AD), which in turn lead into alveolar sacs (AS). A, alveoli; V, blood vessels. × 14.

FIGURE 14-19
Higher-power photomicrograph of part of Figure 14-18 showing an alveolar duct (AD) leading into alveolar sacs (AS). A, alveoli. × 140.

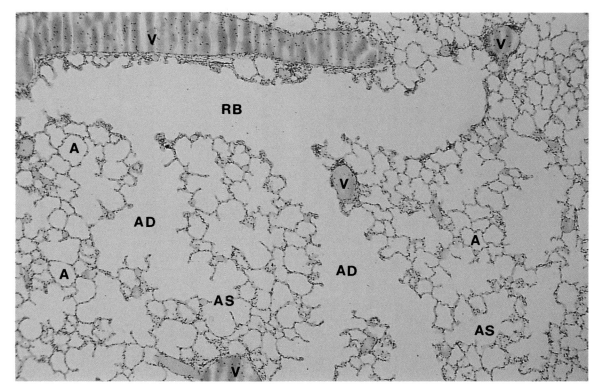

figure 14-18

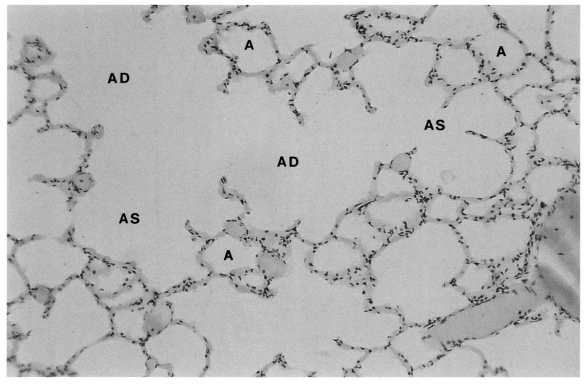

figure 14-19

FIGURE 14-20
Photomicrograph of lung alveolar walls showing squamous (type I) (S) alveolar cells, great (type II) (G) alveolar cells, and alveolar macrophages (M). Note the numerous capillaries (C) in the alveolar wall. A, alveolus. × 869.

FIGURE 14-21
Photomicrograph illustrating intra-alveolar macrophages (arrows). A, alveolus; V, blood vessels. × 560.

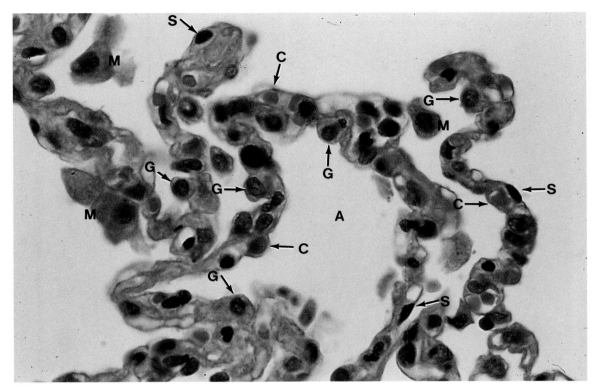

figure 14-20

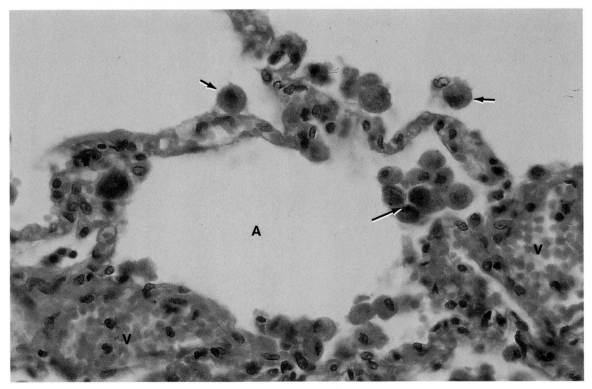

figure 14-21

15 Skin

FIGURE 15-1

Photomicrograph illustrating the stratum corneum (C), stratum granulosum (G), and stratum spinososum (S), and stratum basale (B) of the epidermis and a portion of the underlying dermis (D) of thick skin. × 122.

FIGURE 15-2

Photomicrograph of the epidermis of skin illustrating the change in cellular shape from cuboidal in the stratum basale (B) to squamous in the stratum granulosum (G). Note the spinous processes (arrows) of cells, which form intercellular bridges that are characteristic of the stratum spinosum (S). C, stratum corneum; M, melanocytes. × 487.

FIGURE 15-3

Photomicrograph of thick skin illustrating the stratum lucidum (L) between the stratum corneum (C) and stratum granulosum (G). A small portion of the stratum spinosum (S) is also shown. × 560.

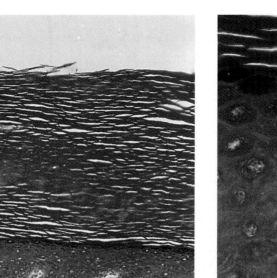

figure 15-1

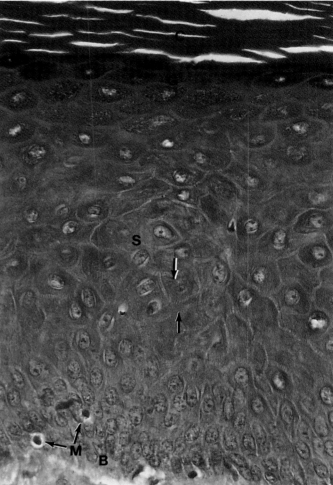

figure 15-2

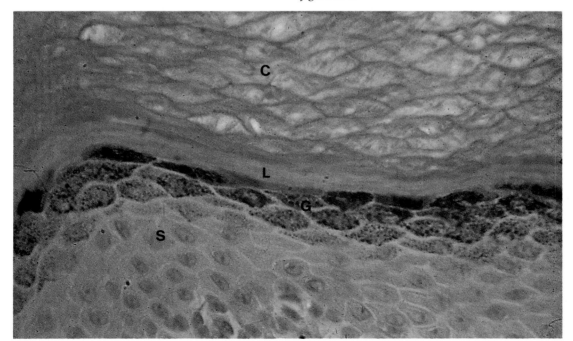

figure 15-3

FIGURE 15-4
Photomicrograph of thin skin. Note the thin stratum corneum (C) and stratum granulo-sum (G). Also shown are the stratum spinosum (S), stratum basale (B), epidermal pegs (EP), dermal papilla (DP), and dermis (D). × 344.

FIGURE 15-5
Photomicrograph of the skin of the scalp showing the epidermis (E), dermis (D), and part of the hypodermis (Hy). Note the hair follicles (H), sebaceous glands (S), and sweat glands (Sg). Two nerve bundles (N) are also shown. × 56.

FIGURE 15-6
Photomicrograph of a sweat gland (Sg), hair follicle (H), and nerve bundle (N) in the dermis of skin. S, secretory portion of the sweat gland; D, duct portion. × 140.

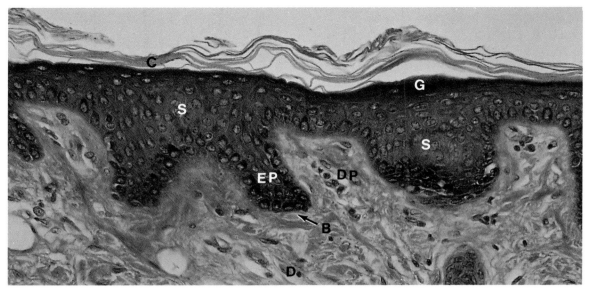

figure 15-4

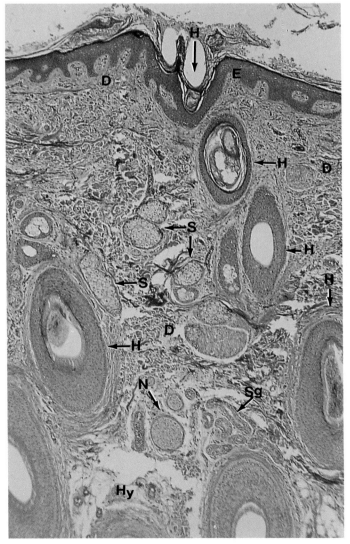

figure 15-5

figure 15-6

FIGURE 15-7
Photomicrograph of a whole mount of a sweat gland. S, secretory portion; D, duct portion. × 5.

FIGURE 15-8
Higher-power photomicrograph of the sweat gland shown in Figure 15-6 illustrating the simple columnar epithelium of the secretory portion (S) of the gland and the stratified cuboidal epithelium of the duct portion (D) of the gland. Note the profiles of nuclei of myoepithelial cells (arrows) in the secretory portion of the gland. BV, blood vessel. × 344.

FIGURE 15-9
Photomicrograph of a sweat gland duct coursing through the stratum spinosum (S), stratum granulosum (G), and stratum corneum (C) of skin. × 430.

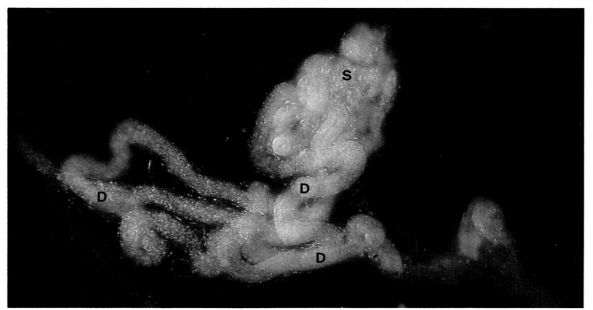

figure 15-7

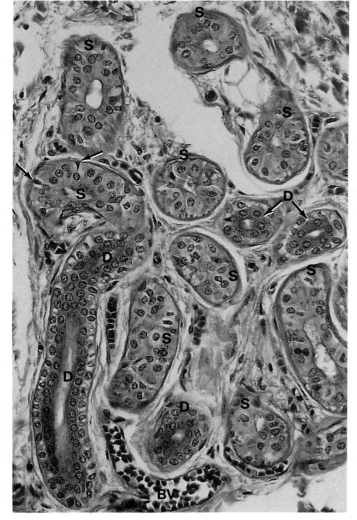

figure 15-8

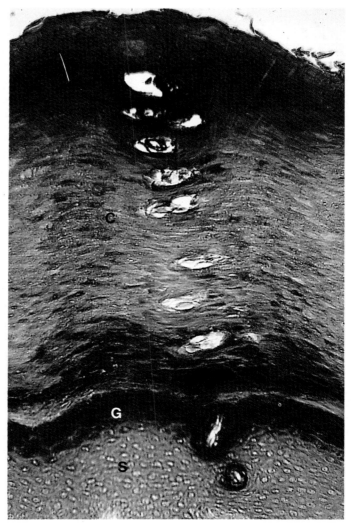

figure 15-9

FIGURE 15-10
Photomicrograph of the acini (S) of a sebaceous gland and its duct (D), which empties into a hair follicle. × 122.

FIGURE 15-11
Photomicrograph of a whole mount of a sebaceous gland fixed in Sudan stain, which stains lipid. × 4.

FIGURE 15-12
Photomicrograph of a whole mount of a sebaceous gland fixed in osmium tetroxide, which stains lipid. × 4.

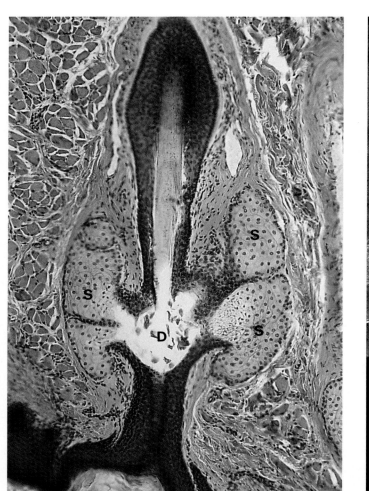

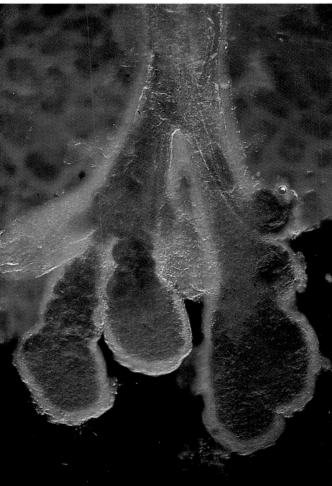

figure 15-10

figure 15-11

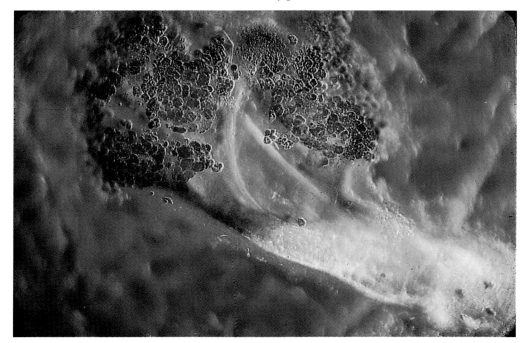

figure 15-12

FIGURE 15-13
Scanning electron micrograph of an oblique section of a hair follicle illustrating its various layers. Shown are the medulla (Me), hair cortex (Co), hair cuticle (Cu), internal root sheath (IRS) (consisting of Henley's layer [He], Huxley's layer [Hu], and the cuticle [CI] of the inner root sheath; CF, collagen fibers), external root sheath (ERS), connective tissue sheath (CTS), and blood vessel (BV). Rabbit; × 2615. (Reprinted with permission from *Tissue and Organs: A Text-Atlas of Scanning Electron Microscopy,* by Richard G. Kessel and Randy H. Kardon. Copyright © 1979 W. H. Freeman & Company.)

FIGURE 15-14
Photomicrograph of a cross section of a hair follicle illustrating the medulla (M), cortex (Co), cuticle (Cu), internal root sheath (IRS), external root sheath (ERS), glassy membrane (G), and connective tissue sheath (CTS). × 140.

FIGURE 15-15
Tangentially cut hair follicle showing the dermal papilla (DP) of the hair bulb and the cortex (Co), internal root sheath (IRS), external root sheath (ERS), glassy membrane (G), and connective tissue sheath (CTS) of the hair follicle. × 140.

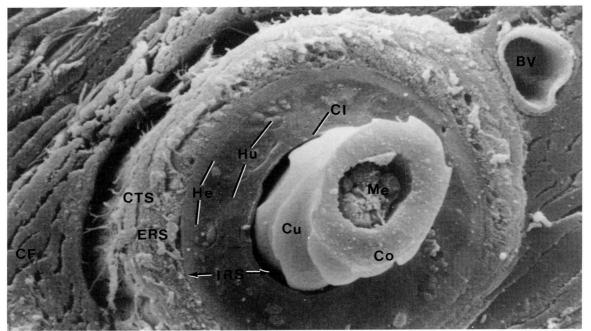

figure 15-13

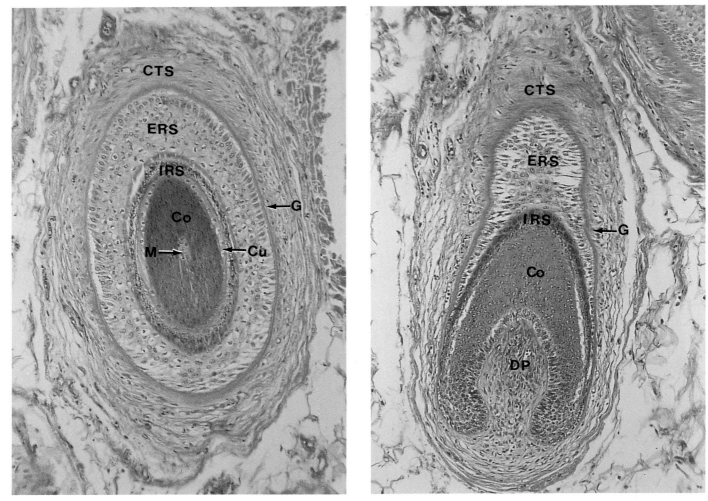

figure 15-14   *figure 15-15*

FIGURE 15-16

Photomicrograph of thin skin of the scalp illustrating melanocytes (arrows) in the stratum basale of the epidermis (E). Also seen are the dermis (D), dermal papillae (DP), epidermal pigs (EP), and blood vessels (V). × 344.

FIGURE 15-17

Higher-power photomicrograph of melanocytes (arrows) in thin skin of the scalp. Note the melanocyte in mitosis (M). E, epidermis; D, dermis; V, blood vessels. × 560.

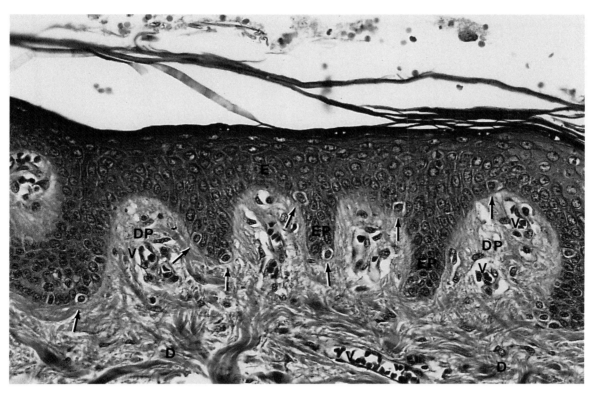

figure 15-16

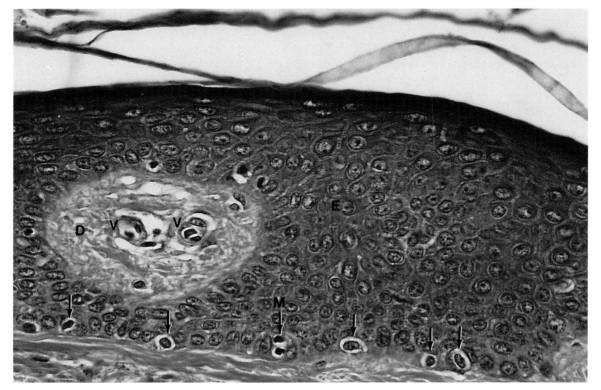

figure 15-17

FIGURE 16-1

Photomicrograph depicting major morphologic features of the kidney: capsule (C), cortex (CO), part of the medulla (M), renal corpuscles (RC), and arcuate blood vessels (A). Note the medullary ray (MR), which is the center of a renal lobule. × 56.

FIGURE 16-2

Photomicrograph of a portion of the cortex (CO) and medulla (M) of the kidney. Note the renal corpuscles (RC) and medullary ray (MR). I, interlobular blood vessels. × 140.

FIGURE 16-3

Photomicrograph of the lower part of the cortex (CO) and upper part of the medulla (M) of the kidney. Note the renal corpuscles (JM) of juxtamedullary nephrons and those of cortical nephrons (RC). A, arcuate blood vessels; I, interlobular blood vessels. × 140.

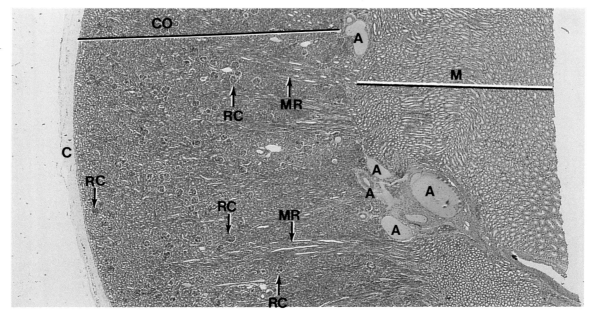

figure 16-1

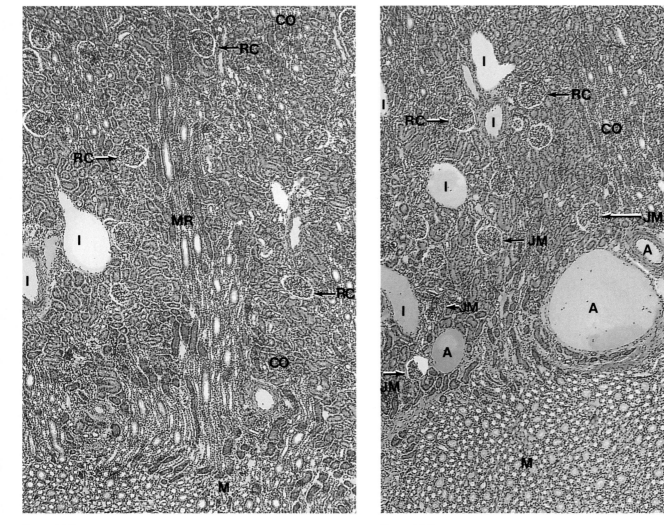

figure 16-2

figure 16-3

FIGURE 16-4
Photomicrograph of the vasculature of the kidney cortex. I, interlobular artery; A, afferent arteriole; G, glomerulus. Injected with carmine. × 125.

FIGURE 16-5
Photomicrograph illustrating an afferent arteriole (A) branching from an interlobular artery (I). The arteriole enters Bowman's capsule and breaks up into a tuft of capillaries forming the glomerulus (G) of a renal corpuscle. × 140.

FIGURE 16-6
Higher-power photomicrograph of the afferent arteriole shown in Figure 16-3. A, afferent arteriole; G, glomerulus; U, urinary space. × 560.

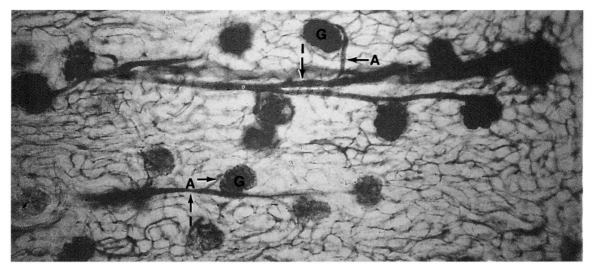

figure 16-4

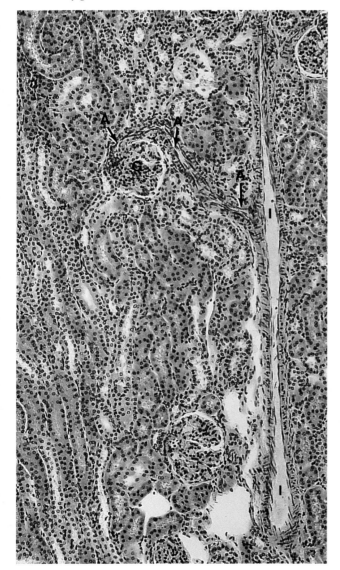

figure 16-5

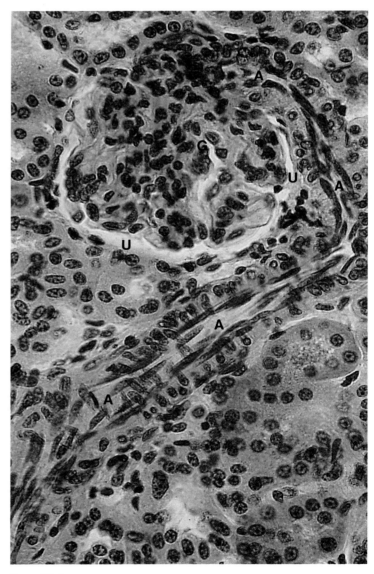

figure 16-6

FIGURE 16-7

Photomicrograph depicting a renal corpuscle of a nephron. Note the simple squamous epithelium of the parietal layer of Bowman's capsule (arrows), which is reflected (bar) at the vascular pole (V) of the nephron, becomes more cuboid, and forms the visceral layer of Bowman's capsule. Visualization of the capillaries of the glomerulus (G) is obscured by visceral epithelial cells (podocytes) and mesangial cells. A, afferent arteriole in cross section; U, urinary space; P, proximal tubules; D, distal tubules. × 560.

FIGURE 16-8

Photomicrograph illustrating the urinary pole of the nephron. The juncture of the parietal layer of Bowman's capsule (arrows) with a proximal convoluted tubule (P) demarcates the urinary pole (UP) of the nephron. Note that the parietal layer of Bowman's capsule is continuous with the epithelium of the proximal tubule, and as it approaches, it becomes more cuboid. The urinary space (U) between the glomerulus (G) and the parietal layer is also continuous with the lumen of the proximal tubule. Apparent are cross-sectioned profiles of proximal (P) and distal (D) tubules. × 560.

FIGURE 16-9

Photomicrograph illustrating the macula densa (arrows), which are modified cells of the distal convoluted tubule (DCT), one component of the juxtaglomerular apparatus, and the afferent arteriole (A), whose modified smooth muscle cells are a second component of the juxtaglomerular apparatus. Also apparent is a glomerulus (G), with its urinary space (U). P, proximal convoluted tubules; A, thick ascending (distal) tubules. × 560.

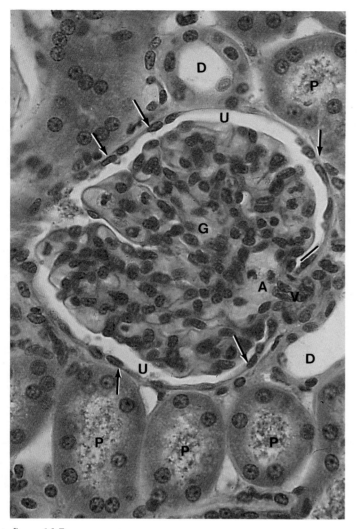

figure 16-7

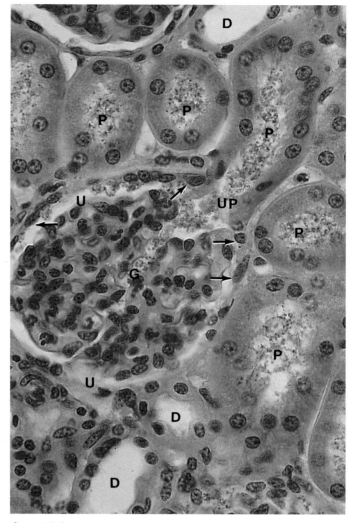

figure 16-8

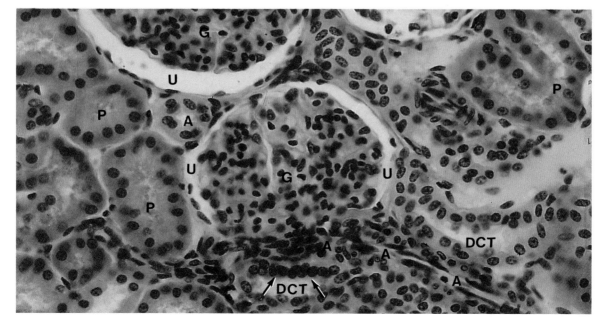

figure 16-9

FIGURE 16-10

Scanning electron micrograph of podocytes, the visceral epithelial cells of Bowman's capsule. Shown are the cell body (CB) and the primary branch (PB) and secondary branch (SB) for podocyte cell processes. × 5325. (Reprinted with permission from *Tissue and Organs: A Text-Atlas of Scanning Electron Microscopy*, by Richard G. Kessel and Randy H. Kardon. W. H. Freeman & Company, 1979.)

FIGURE 16-11

Electron micrograph of the filtration barrier of a renal corpuscle. Shown are the urinary space (US), pedicels (PE), and filtration slits (FS). Note the three components of the basal lamina (BL), the lamina rara interna (LRI), lamina densa (LD), and lamina rara externa (LRE). CL, capillary lumen; E, capillary endothelium; F, fenestration of the endothelium. Mouse; × 61,750. (Courtesy of Dr. Richard L. Wood.)

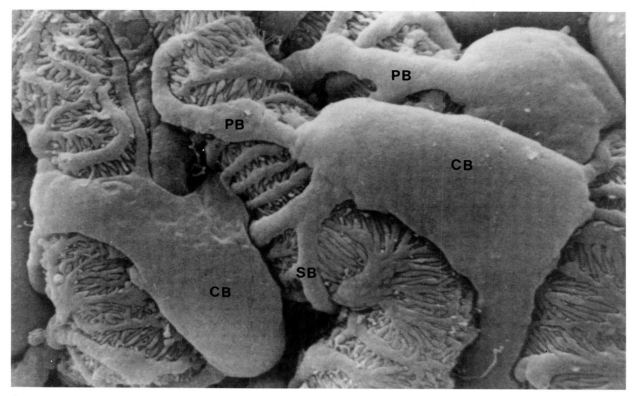

figure 16-10

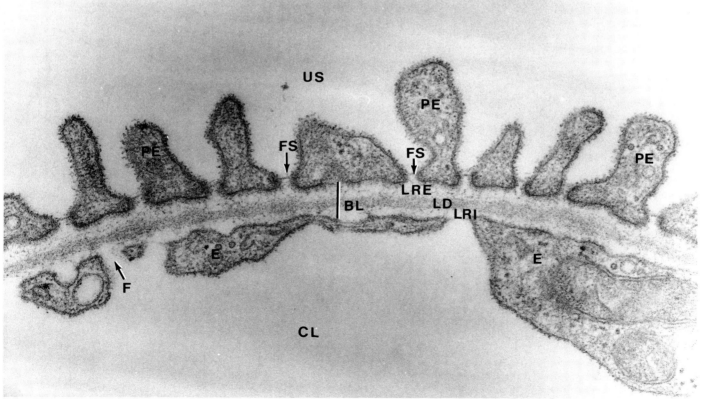

figure 16-11

FIGURE 16-12
Photomicrograph of cross-sectioned tubules in the kidney medulla. D, thick descending (proximal) tubules; A, thick ascending (distal) tubules; T, collecting tubules. × 344.

FIGURE 16-13
Photomicrograph of longitudinally sectioned collecting tubules (CT). Note the distinct lateral cell boundaries (arrows) between the cuboidal epithelial cells. × 344.

FIGURE 16-14
Photomicrograph of a collecting duct (CD), thin limb (TL) of the loop of Henle, and vasa rectae (V). Note the distinct cell boundaries (arrows) of the simple columnar epithelium of the duct. × 344.

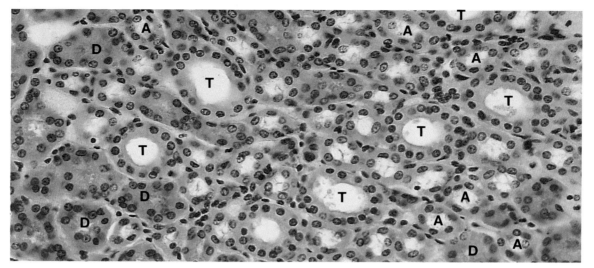

figure 16-12

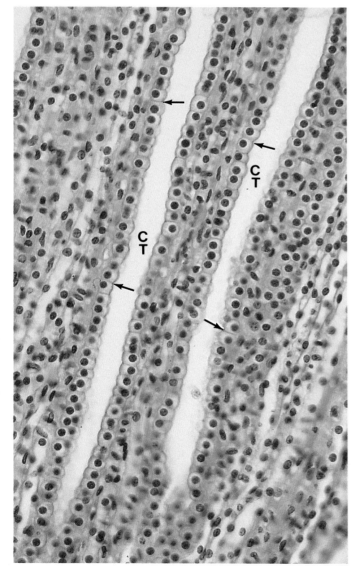

figure 16-13

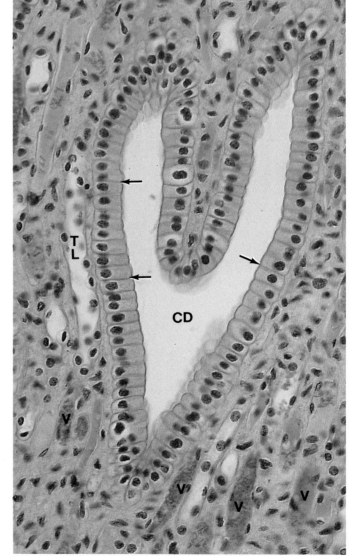

figure 16-14

FIGURE 16-15
Photomicrograph of the apex of a medullary pyramid. The epithelium (E) of the apex is transitional, as is the epithelium of the minor calyx (EC) into which urine is emptied. C, space of the minor calyx; DB, ducts of Bellini; V, vasa rectae; CD, collecting ducts. × 49.

FIGURE 16-16
Photomicrograph of a ureter in a relaxed state cut in cross section. Note the convoluted nature of the mucosa, consisting of transitional epithelium (T) and underlying lamina propria (LP). The muscularis is organized in poorly demarcated inner longitudinal (IL) and outer circular (OC) layers of smooth muscle. A, adventitia; F, fat. × 49.

FIGURE 16-17
Higher-power photomicrograph of a portion of Figure 16-16 illustrating the transitional epithelium (T) and lamina propria (LP) of the mucosa and the inner longitudinal (IL) and outer circular (OC) smooth muscle of the muscularis. × 122.

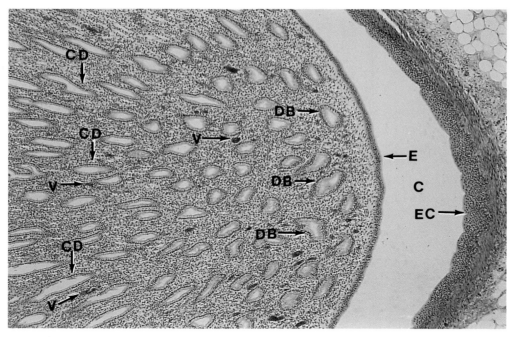

figure 16-15

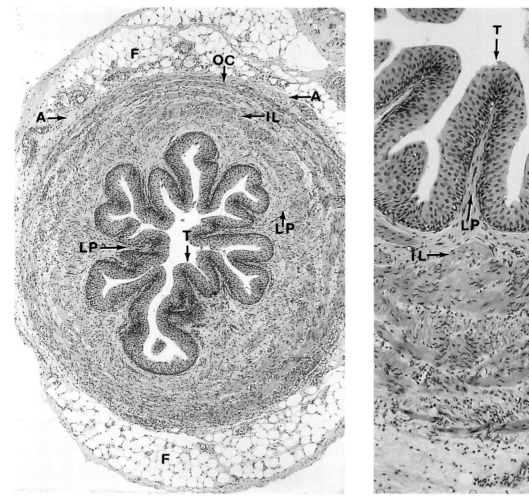

figure 16-16

figure 16-17

FIGURE 16-18
Photomicrograph of the urinary bladder. Note the thick muscularis arranged as inner longitudinal (IL), middle circular (MC), and outer longitudinal (OL) layers. T, transitional epithelium; LP, lamina propria; A, adventitia. × 14.

FIGURE 16-19
Higher-power photomicrograph of a portion of Figure 16-18. Note the transitional epithelium (T), lumen (L), and lamina propria (LP) of the mucosa of the bladder. A part of the inner longitudinal (IL) muscle layer is shown. × 56.

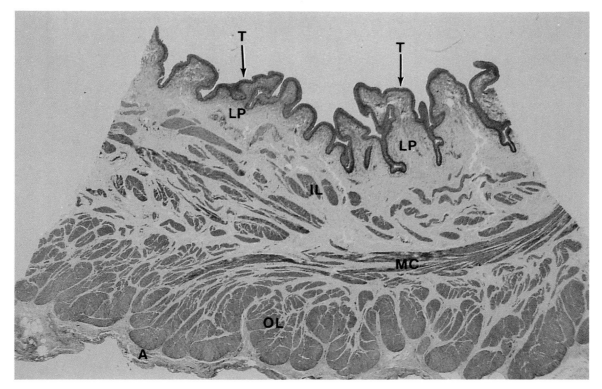

figure 16-18

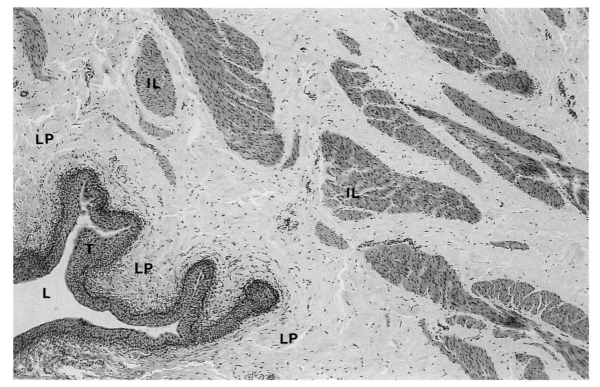

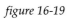

figure 16-19

FIGURE 17-1

Photomicrograph illustrating the pars distalis (PD), pars intermedia (PI), pars nervosa (PN), and pars tuberalis (PT) of the hypophysis or pituitary gland. × 14.

FIGURE 17-2

Photomicrograph depicting basophils (B) and acidophils (A), the chromophilic cells of the pars distalis, or anterior lobe, of the pituitary gland. Note the blood sinuses (S). × 344.

FIGURE 17-3

Photomicrograph illustrating basophils (B), acidophils (A), and chromophobe cells (C) of the anterior lobe of the pituitary gland. S, sinusoid. × 560.

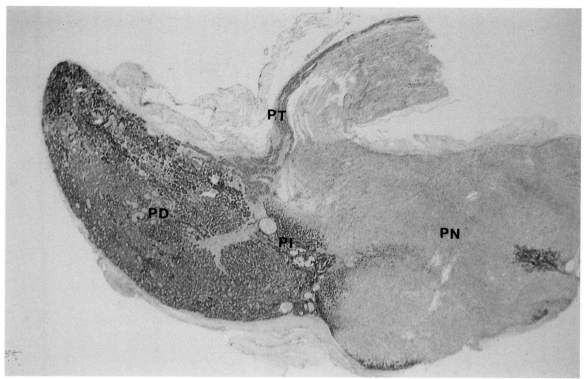

figure 17-1

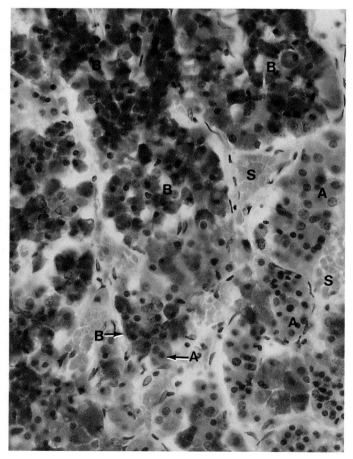

figure 17-2

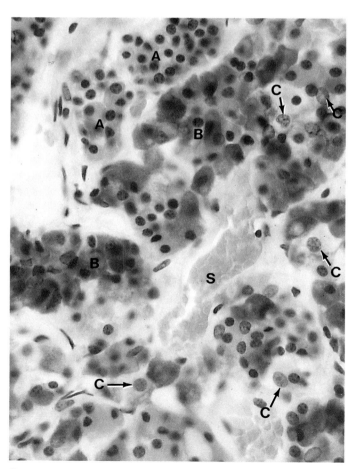

figure 17-3

FIGURE 17-4
Photomicrograph of the pituitary gland illustrating Rathke's cysts (C) in the intermediate lobe (PI) of the pituitary gland and incursion of basophils (B) into the pars nervosa (PN). PD, pars distalis. × 56.

FIGURE 17-5
Higher-power photomicrograph of a portion of Figure 17-4 depicting basophils (B) of the intermediate lobe in the pars nervosa (PN). The unmyelinated axons of hypothalamic neurons which comprise the bulk of the pars nervosa are not readily distinguished in hematoxylin-and-eosin-stained material. The nuclei of most cells seen in this micrograph are those of pituicytes (glial cells), which act as support cells for the unmyelinated axons. × 56.

FIGURE 17-6
Photomicrograph depicting pituicytes of the pars nervosa, some of which (arrows) contain lipofuscin. × 560.

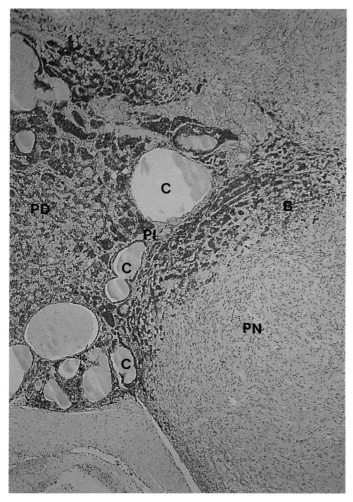

figure 17-4

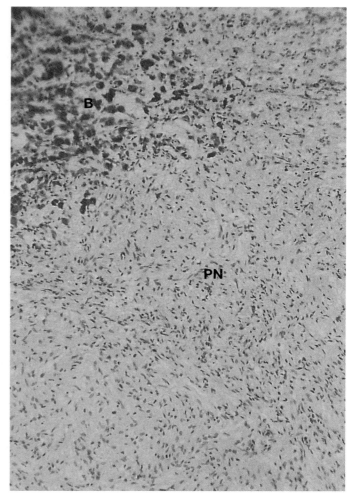

figure 17-5

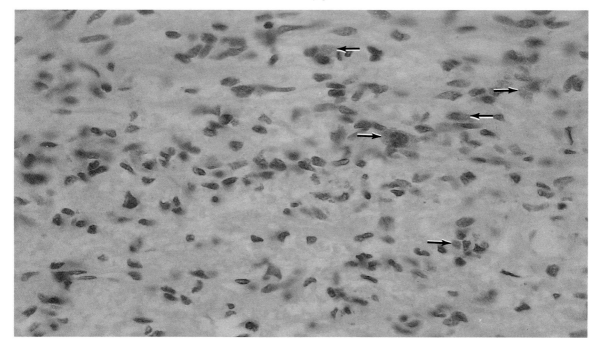

figure 17-6

FIGURE 17-7
Photomicrograph of the adrenal gland illustrating the cortex (Co), the medulla (M), the capsule (C), and venous blood vessels (V) in the medulla of the gland. × 14.

FIGURE 17-8
Photomicrograph depicting four morphologically distinct parts: the zona glomerulosa (G), zona fasciculata (F), zona reticularis (R), and medulla (M) of the adrenal cortex. C, capsule. × 140.

FIGURE 17-9
Photomicrograph illustrating the adrenal medulla (M) surrounded by cells of the zona reticularis (R). V, veins. × 56.

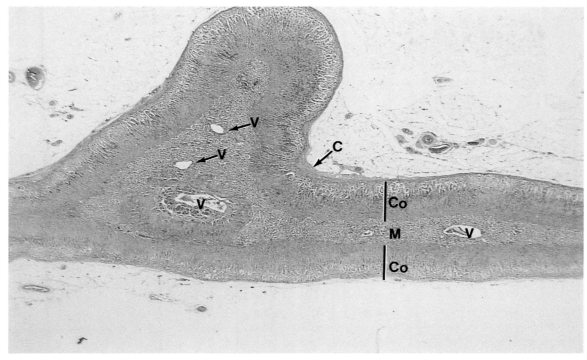

figure 17-7

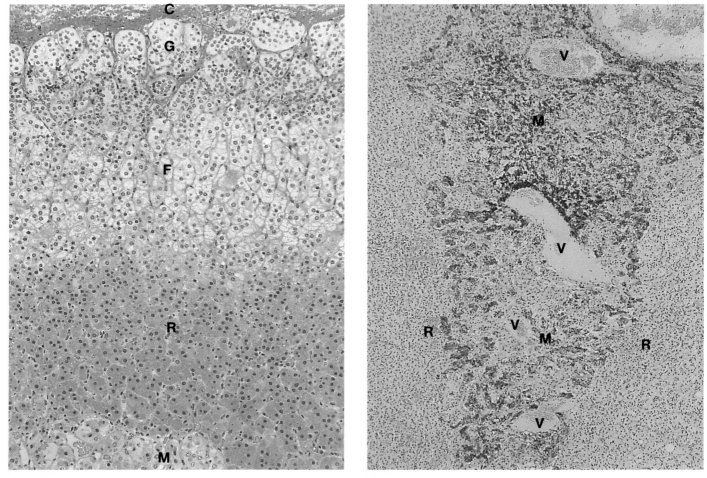

figure 17-8

figure 17-9

FIGURE 17-10

Photomicrograph emphasizing the morphologic difference between the zona reticularis (R) and the medulla (M) of the adrenal gland. V, vein. × 140.

FIGURE 17-11

Photomicrograph illustrating the cells of the adrenal medulla, all of which do not stain with the same intensity. Note the ganglion cell (G), which is not uncommon to the medulla. × 560.

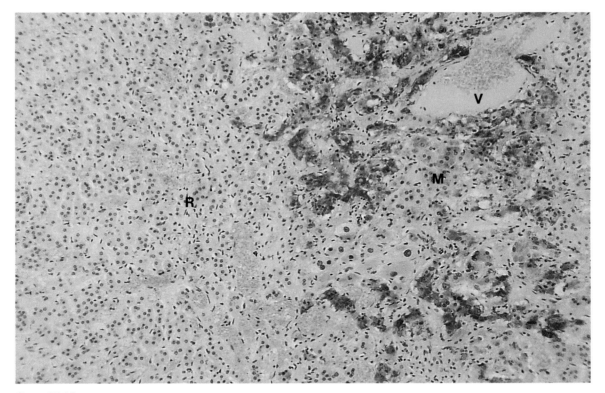

figure 17-10

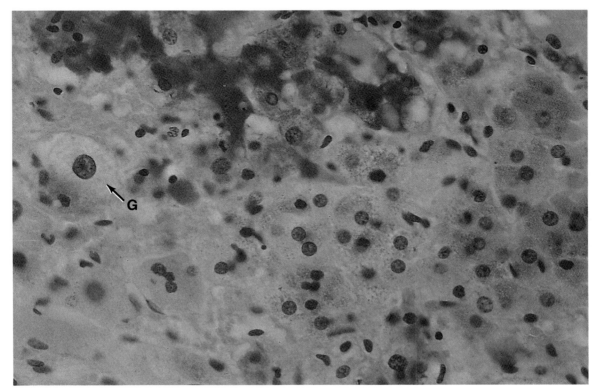

figure 17-11

FIGURE 17-12
Photomicrograph of the pancreas depicting the islets of Langerhans (arrows), the endocrine portion of the gland. × 56.

FIGURE 17-13
Photomicrograph emphasizing the morphologic difference between the endocrine cells of an islet of Langerhans (IL) and surrounding serous acinar cells of the exocrine portion of the pancreas. × 344.

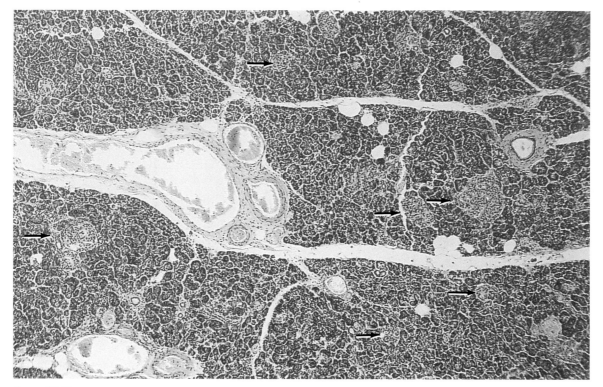

figure 17-12

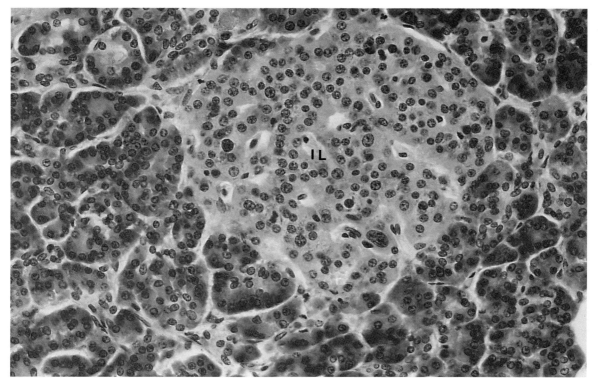

figure 17-13

FIGURE 17-14
Photomicrograph of the thyroid gland. The follicles, containing pink-staining colloid, are the functional units of the gland. C, capsule of the gland. × 56.

FIGURE 17-15
Photomicrograph of thyroid follicles (F) showing pink-stained colloid within the follicles and the simple cuboidal epithelium that lines the follicle. Note the parafollicular, or "C," cell (C). × 344.

FIGURE 17-16
Photomicrograph illustrating the parafollicular, or "C," cells (C) of the thyroid. F, follicles with colloid; A, arteriole. × 560.

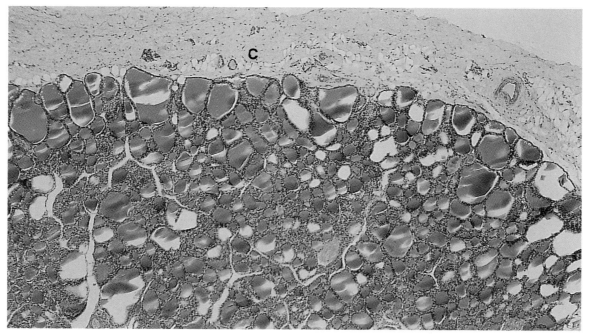

figure 17-14

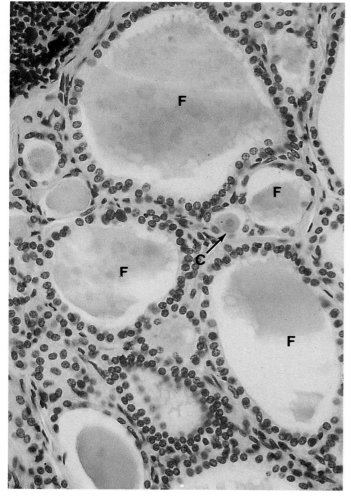

figure 17-15

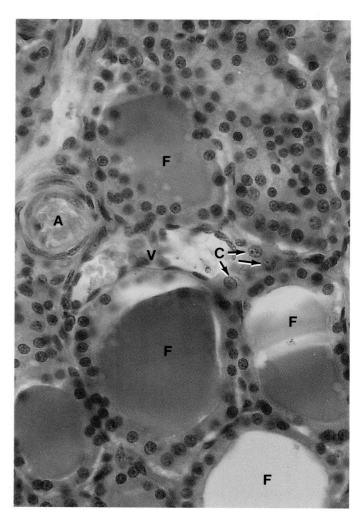

figure 17-16

FIGURE 17-17
Photomicrograph of the parathyroid gland illustrating chief cells (C) and a large group of oxyphil cells (O). × 56.

FIGURE 17-18
Photomicrograph illustrating interstitial cells of Leydig (L), the hormone-secreting cells of the testis. Note the close proximity of the Leydig cells to blood vessels (V). × 344.

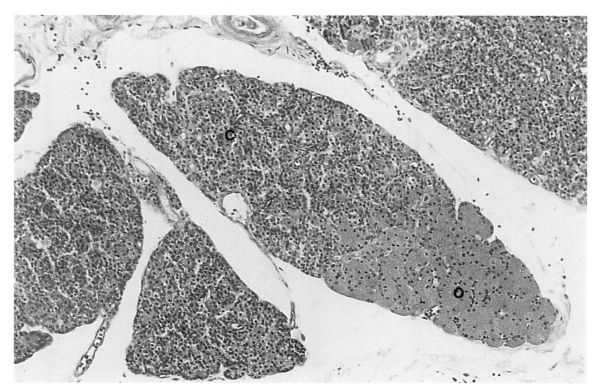

figure 17-17

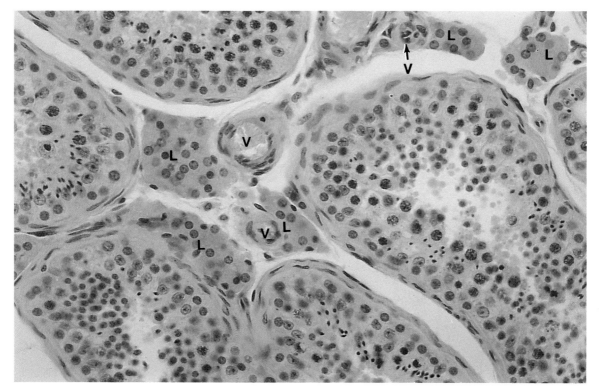

figure 17-18

FIGURE 17-19

Photomicrograph of a secondary ovarian follicle, a temporary endocrine organ. The granulosa cells (G) of the follicle secrete estrogen during the first half, or preovulatory, stage of the menstrual cycle. After ovulation, the granulosa cells in conjunction with theca interna cells form another temporary endocrine gland, the corpus luteum. Dog; × 344.

FIGURE 17-20

Photomicrograph of a portion of a corpus luteum composed of granulosa lutein and theca lutein cells, which secrete progesterone and estrogen during the second half, or postovulatory, stage of the menstrual cycle. If pregnancy does not occur, the corpus luteum ceases functioning. If pregnancy occurs, the corpus luteum persists for approximately six months and continues secreting progesterone and estrogen. Dog; × 56.

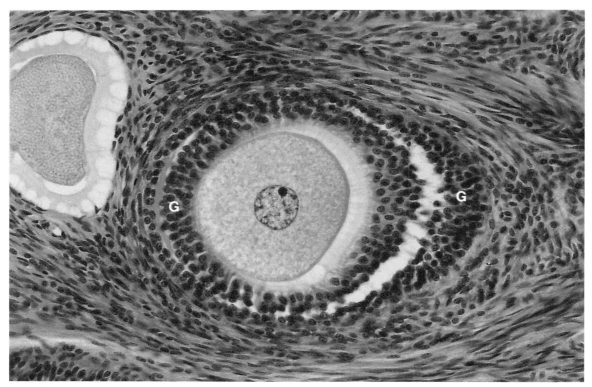

figure 17-19

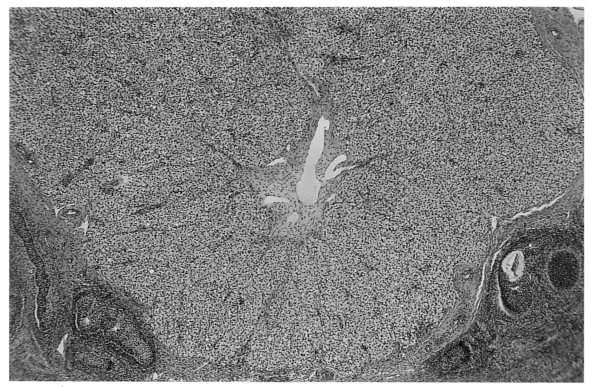

figure 17-20

FIGURE 18-1

Photomicrograph of the testis, epididymis (E), and part of the ductus deferens (D). Note the tunica albuginea (AL), which on the posterior surface of the testis becomes thickened and forms the mediastinum testes (M). Note also the connective tissue septae (arrows), which divide the testis into lobules containing the seminiferous tubules (S). R, rete testis. The spaces labeled A are artifacts of fixation. × 14.

FIGURE 18-2

Photomicrograph of part of the testis showing profiles of seminiferous tubules (S) and the rete testes (R) within the mediastinum (M). × 56.

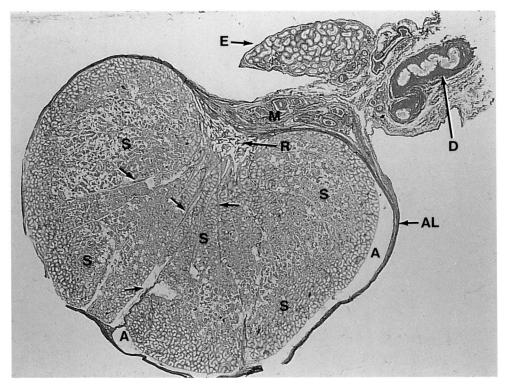

figure 18-1

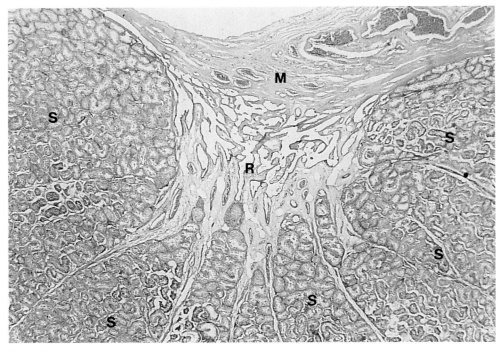

figure 18-2

FIGURE 18-3

Photomicrograph of transverse sections of seminiferous tubules from an inactive testis. Note the paucity of developing cellular elements in the tubular epithelium. Sg, spermatogonia; Ps, primary spermatocytes; St, spermatids; Sc, sertoli cells; BM, basement membrane. × 222.

FIGURE 18-4

Photomicrograph illustrating the different cellular associations in the seminiferous epithelium of seminiferous tubules in an active testis. Sg, spermatogonia; Ps, primary spermatocytes; St, early spermatids; Lst, late spermatids; Sc, Sertoli cells; L, interstitial cells of Leydig. × 299.

FIGURE 18-5

Photomicrograph of parts of seminiferous tubules illustrating spermatogonia (Sg) and spermatogonia in mitosis (arrows). Note the primary spermatocytes (Ps) and the Sertoli (Sc), myoid (M), and fibroblast (F) cells. CT, connective tissue; L, interstitial cells of Leydig. × 487.

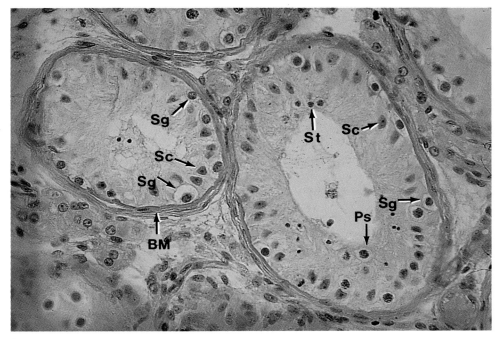

figure 18-3

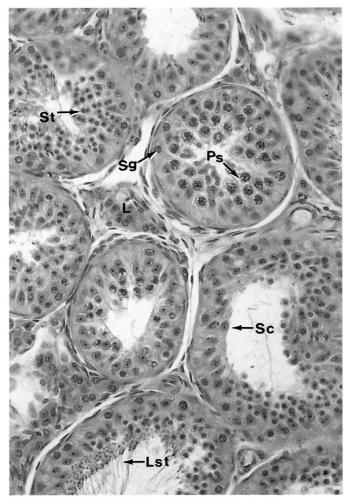

figure 18-4

figure 18-5

FIGURE 18-6
High-power photomicrograph of a seminiferous tubule showing spermatogonia (Sg), primary spermatocytes (Ps), early spermatids (St), and Sertoli cells (Sc) in the epithelium. Note the nuclei of myoid cells (M) and fibroblasts (F) of the tubule. Monkey; × 756.

FIGURE 18-7
Photomicrograph of a seminiferous tubule showing a preponderance of primary spermatocytes (Ps) in its epithelium. Note the spermatogonia (Sg) and the myoid (M) and fibroblast (F) cell nuclei. A prominent basement membrane (BM) is also evident. Monkey; × 756.

FIGURE 18-8
Photomicrograph of a seminiferous tubule in which late spermatids (Lst) and Sertoli cells (Sc) are the predominant cell types in the epithelium. Note the spermatogonia (Sg), primary spermatocytes (Ps), and early spermatids (St). BM, basement membrane; M, myoid cell nucleus; F, fibroblast nucleus. Monkey; × 756.

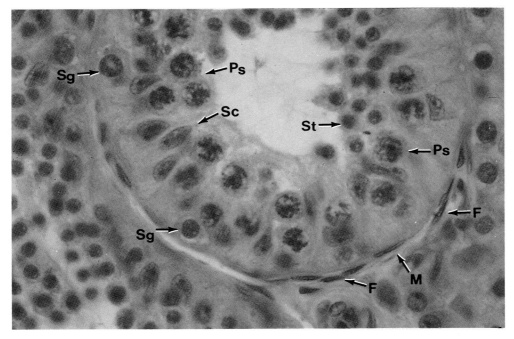

figure 18-6

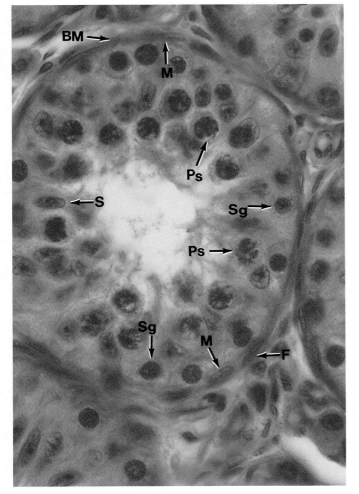

figure 18-7

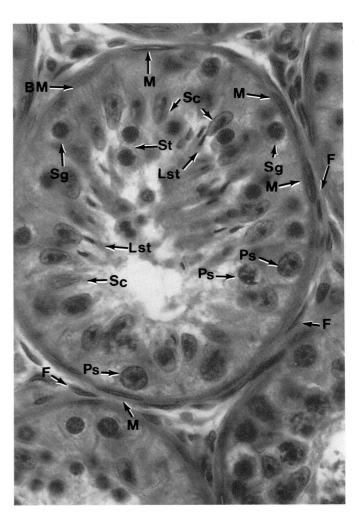

figure 18-8

FIGURE 18-9
Photomicrograph illustrating seminiferous tubules (S), the rete testes (R) in the connective tissue (CT) of the mediastinum, and a portion of an efferent duct (E). × 42.

FIGURE 18-10
Photomicrograph showing a seminiferous tubule (S) leading into a tubulus rectus (Tr), which in turn joins the rete testes (R). Note the numerous blood vessels (V) in the connective tissue (CT) of the mediastinum. × 122.

FIGURE 18-11
Higher-power photomicrograph of a portion of Figure 18-10 illustrating the very short tubulus rectus (Tr), which joins the seminiferous tubule (S) to the rete testis (R). × 487.

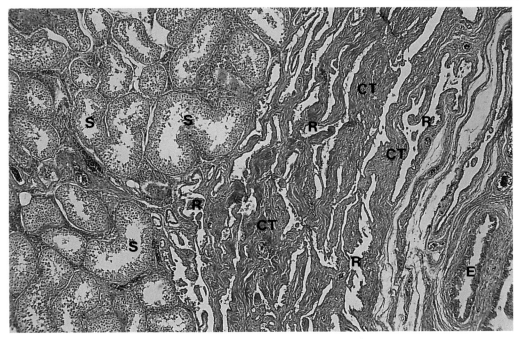

figure 18-9

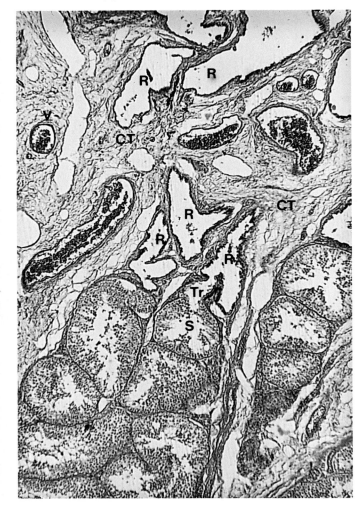

figure 18-10

figure 18-11

FIGURE 18-12

Photomicrograph illustrating the junction (arrows) of the rete testis (R) with an efferent duct (Ef). Note the profiles of other efferent ducts (E), the connective tissue (CT), and blood vessels (V) of the mediastinum. × 56.

FIGURE 18-13

Photomicrograph of an efferent tubule showing the uneven or scalloped nature of its epithelium, which is characteristic of the tubule. Some of the epithelial cells are ciliated (arrows). CT, connective tissue; V, blood vessels. × 344.

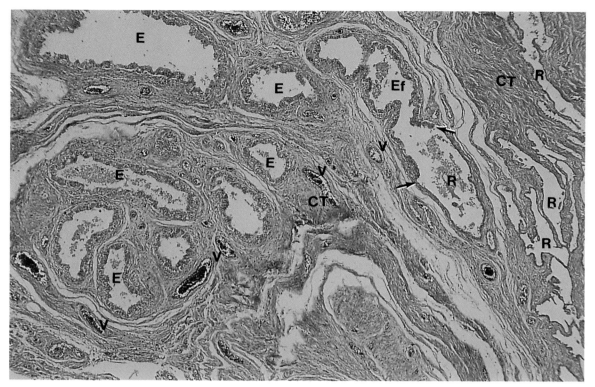

figure 18-12

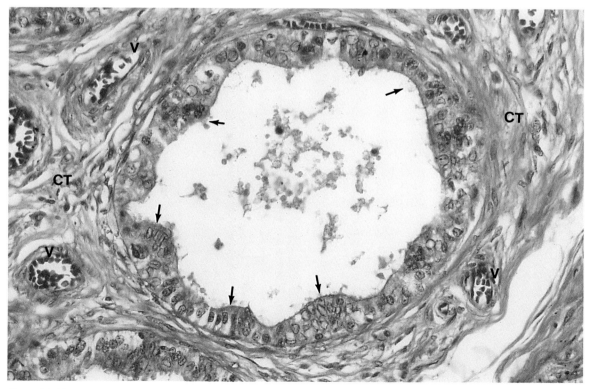

figure 18-13

FIGURE 18-14
Photomicrograph of the ductus epididymis showing the variety of profiles obtained when this single highly convoluted tubule is cut in cross section. Note the smooth appearance of the steriociliated epithelium (arrows). Sz, spermatozoa; V, blood vessels. × 140.

FIGURE 18-15
High-power photomicrograph of a portion of the ductus epididymis. The pseudo-stratified columnar epithelium (bar) has prominent basal cells (arrows) and stereocilia (Sc). Sz, spermatozoa; SM, smooth muscle. × 344.

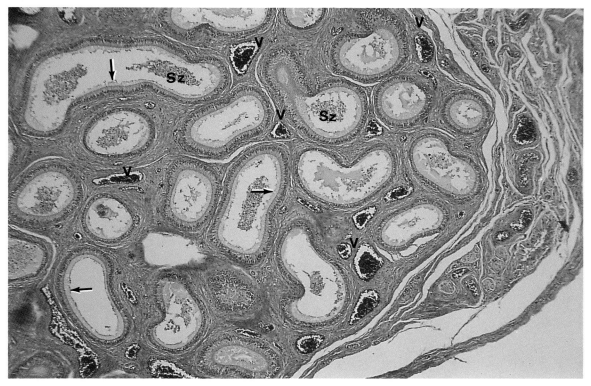

figure 18-14

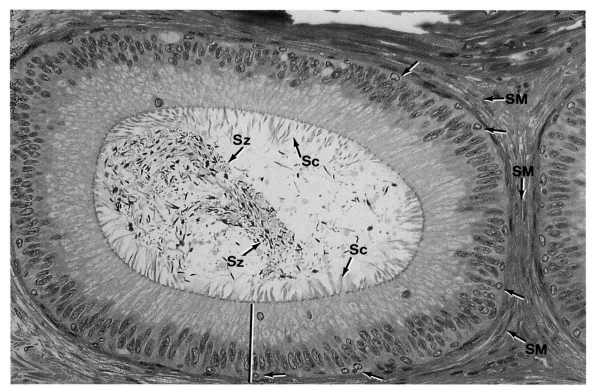

figure 18-15

FIGURE 18-16
Photomicrograph of the ductus (vas) deferens. Note the thick muscularis composed of inner longitudinal (IL), middle circular (MC), and outer longitudinal (OL) layers of smooth muscle. E, pseudostratified epithelium; LP, lamina propria; A, adventitia. × 56.

FIGURE 18-17
Higher-power photomicrograph of the ductus (vas) deferens. Its mucosa is composed of pseudostratified columnar epithelium (E) with stereocilia (arrow) and a lamina propria (LP). Parts of the inner longitudinal (IL) and middle circular (MC) smooth muscle cell layers are also shown. × 140.

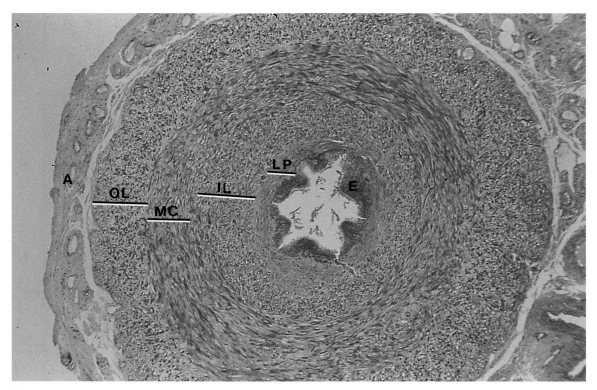

figure 18-16

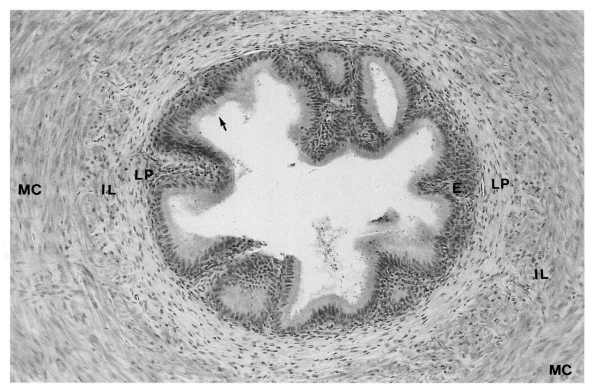

figure 18-17

FIGURE 18-18
Photomicrograph of the seminal vesicle illustrating the highly folded nature of its mucosa (arrows). The folds project into and seemingly compartmentalize the single lumen (L) of the organ. × 14.

FIGURE 18-19
Photomicrograph illustrating the branched and highly folded mucosa of the seminal vesicle. Note the epithelium (arrows) and lamina propria (LP) of the mucosa. The lumen (L) of the organ appears compartmentalized by folds of the mucosa. Note also the thick muscular layer (M) beneath the mucosa. × 140.

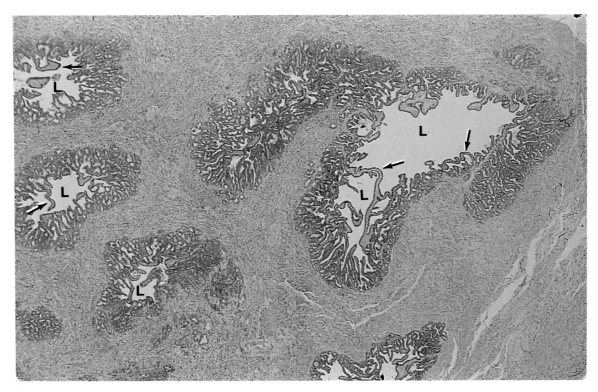

figure 18-18

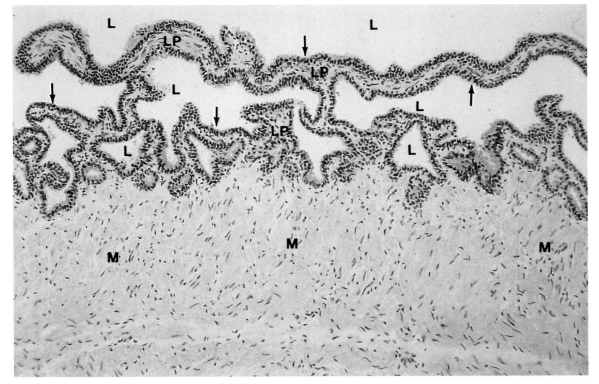

figure 18-19

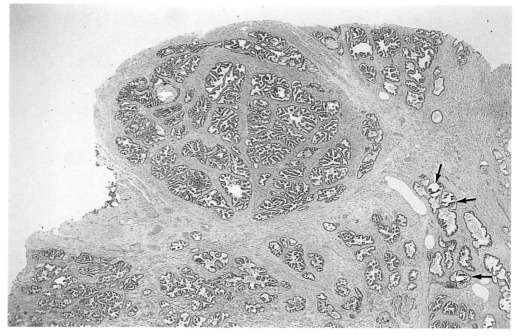

figure 18-20

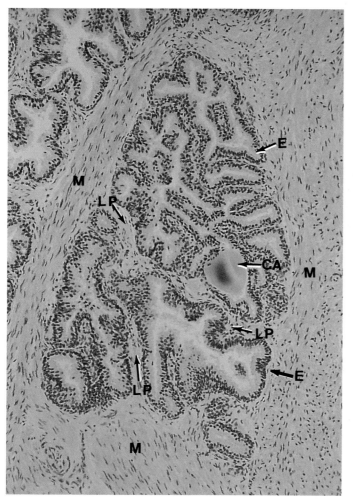

figure 18-21

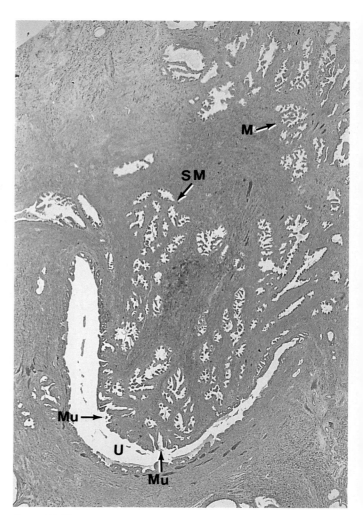

figure 18-22

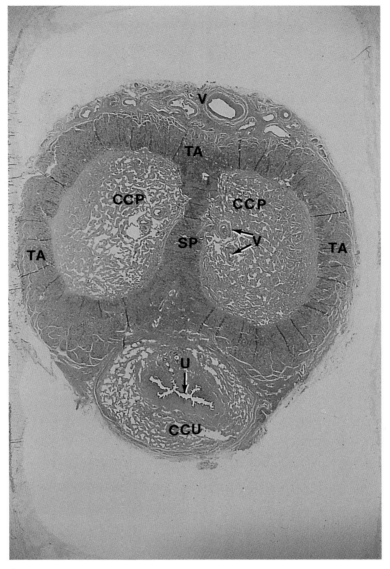

figure 18-23

FIGURE 18-20
Photomicrograph of the tubuloalveolar glands of the prostate. Note the prostatic concretions, or corpora amylacea (arrows). × 12.

FIGURE 18-21
Higher-power photomicrograph of a portion of the prostate shown in Figure 18-20. Note the convoluted epithelium (E), the lamina propria (LP), a prostatic concretion (CA), and smooth muscle (M) of the surrounding stromal tissue. × 122.

FIGURE 18-22
Photomicrograph of the prostate illustrating the prostatic urethra (U), mucosal glands emptying into the urethra (Mu), submucosal glands (SM), and main glands (M). × 12.

FIGURE 18-23
Photomicrograph of a transverse section of the penis. U, urethra; CCU, corpus cavernosum urethra; CCP, corpus cavernosum penis; TA, tunica albuginea; SP, septum penis; V, blood vessels. × 5.

19 The Female Reproductive System

FIGURE 19-1

Photomicrograph of an ovary illustrating the tunica albuginea (A) and the cortex (C) with follicles (F) in various stages of development. The medulla (M) of the ovary is well vascularized (V). Note the corpus luteum (CL) and germinal epithelium (arrows), which is a misnomer. Dog; × 14.

FIGURE 19-2

Photomicrograph of primordial (P) and unilaminar primary (UF) follicles. O, oocyte; G, granulosa (follicular) cells. Dog; × 344.

FIGURE 19-3

Photomicrograph of primordial (P), unilaminar primary (UF), and multilaminar primary (MF) follicles. Note the zona pellucida (arrow) in the multilaminar primary follicle. O, oocyte; G, granulosa (follicular) cells. × 344.

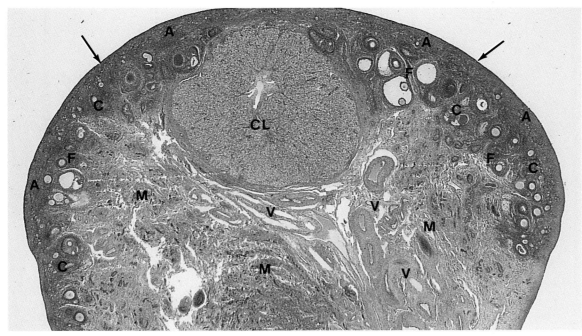

figure 19-1

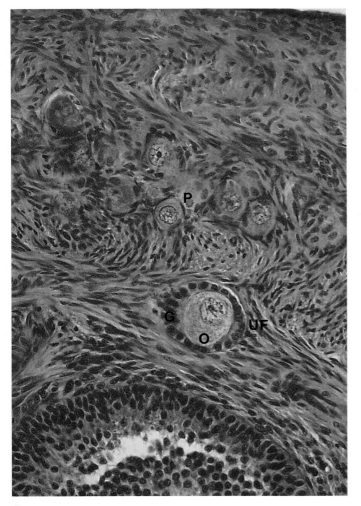

figure 19-2

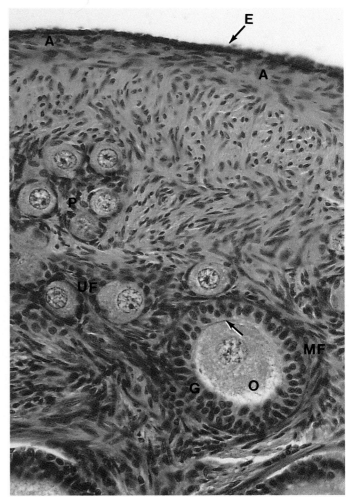

figure 19-3

FIGURE 19-4
Photomicrograph of a multilaminar primary follicle. Note the mitotic figure (unlabeled arrow) in the granulosa cell layer (G). Note the cuboidal cells of the theca interna (TI). O, oocyte; Z, zona pellucida. Dog; × 560.

FIGURE 19-5
Photomicrograph contrasting a unilaminar primary follicle (UF) and a well-developed multilaminar primary follicle (MF). Note the thickness of the granulosa cell layer (G) in the multilaminar primary follicle and the basement membrane (b) separating the granulosa from the developing theca folliculi (TF). O, oocyte; Z, zona pellucida. Dog; × 344.

FIGURE 19-6
Photomicrograph contrasting a multilaminar primary follicle (MF) and an early secondary follicle (SF). Note in particular the presence of an antrum (A) in the secondary follicle, which distinguishes secondary from primary follicles. Note also the mitotic figure (arrow) and thick theca folliculi (bar) of the secondary follicle. O, oocyte; b, basement membrane; Z, zona pellucida; G, granulosa cell layer. Dog; × 344.

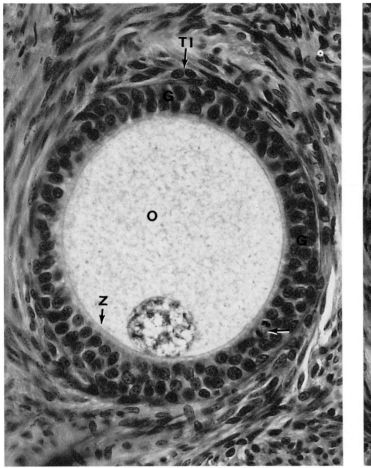

figure 19-4

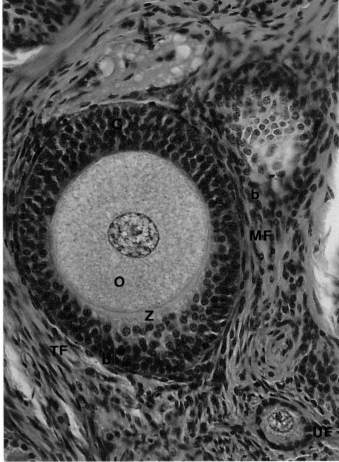

figure 19-5

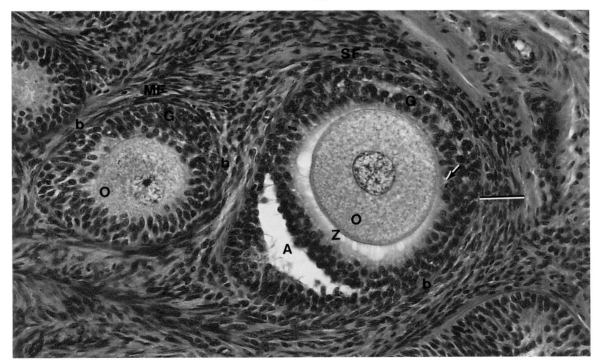

figure 19-6

FIGURE 19-7
Photomicrograph contrasting a Graafian (GF) and a secondary (SF) follicle. Note the corona radiata (CR), the single layer of granulosa cells that are in immediate contact with the zona pellucida (z) and remain with the ovum after ovulation. O, oocyte; bar, theca folliculi; A, antrum. Dog; × 140.

FIGURE 19-8
Photomicrograph of a corpus albicans, the dense connective tissue remnant resulting from the functional regression and involution of a corpus luteum (see Figure 19-1). × 56.

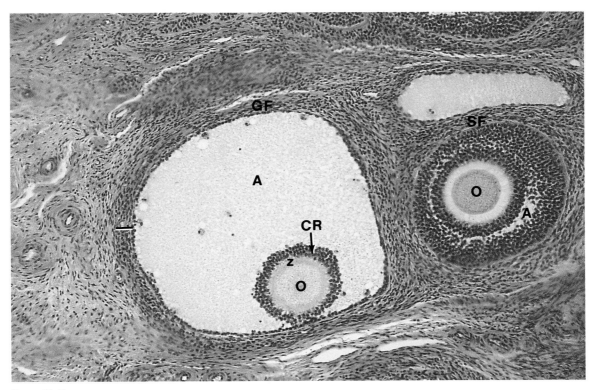

figure 19-7

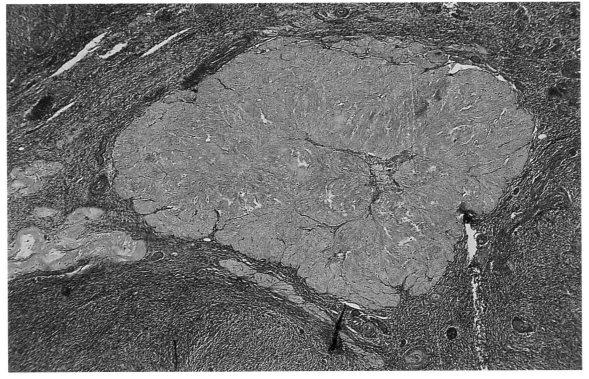

figure 19-8

FIGURE 19-9
Photomicrograph of an atretic early secondary follicle. O, oocyte; G, degenerating granulosa cells. Dog; × 140.

FIGURE 19-10
Photomicrograph contrasting a normal secondary follicle (SF) with an atretic late secondary follicle (ASF). G, degenerating granulosa cells; O, oocyte; Z, zona pellucida; A, antrum. Dog; × 140.

FIGURE 19-11
Photomicrograph of an atretic primary follicle. Note persisting zona pellucida (Z). G, degenerating granulosa cells; O, oocyte. Dog; × 344.

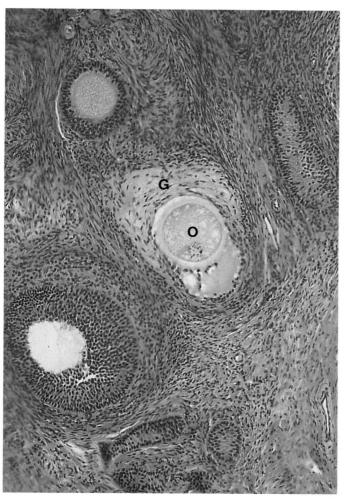

figure 19-9

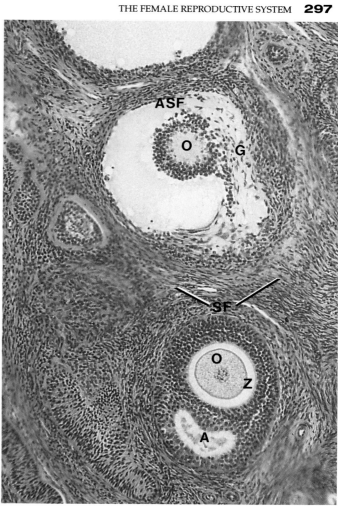

figure 19-10

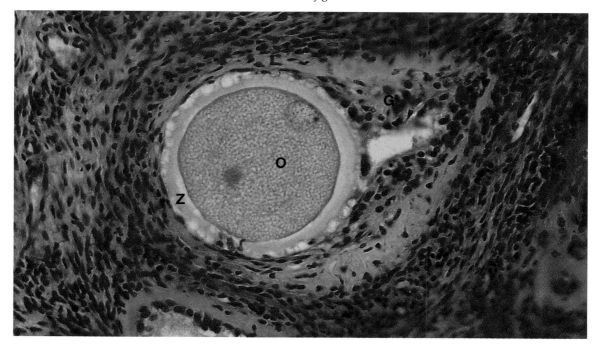

figure 19-11

FIGURE 19-12
Photomicrograph illustrating the fimbriated (F) and ampullatory (A) portions of the oviduct. BL, broad ligament; O, ovary; SF, secondary follicle; arrows, blood vessels in the broad ligament. Masson's stain. Cat; × 56.

FIGURE 19-13
Photomicrograph illustrating the isthmus (I) of the oviduct (which because of folding during tissue preparation shows three profiles) in relation to the broad ligament (BL). O, ovary; SF, secondary follicle; arrows, blood vessels of the broad ligament. Masson's stain. Cat; × 56.

FIGURE 19-14
Photomicrograph illustrating the epithelium (E), lamina propria (LP), and muscularis (M) of the isthmus of the oviduct. BL, broad ligament; arrows, blood vessels. Masson's stain. Cat; × 140.

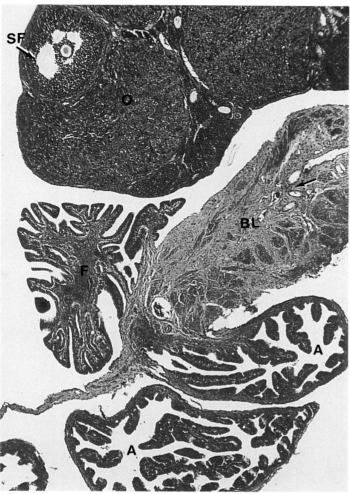

figure 19-12

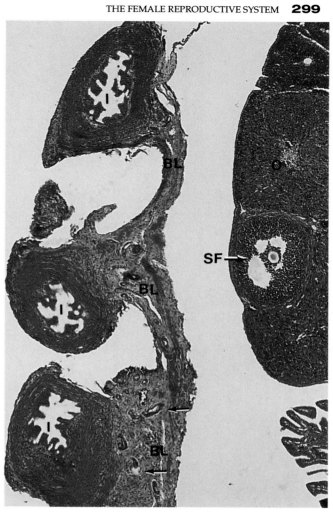

figure 19-13

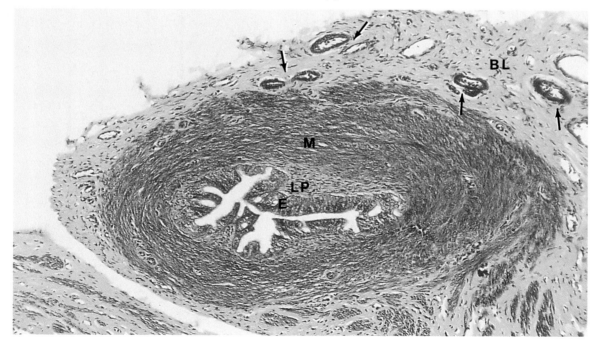

figure 19-14

FIGURE 19-15

Photomicrograph contrasting the ampulla (A) and isthmus (I) of the oviduct, which because of folding during tissue preparation appear in the same section. BL, broad ligament. × 14.

FIGURE 19-16

Photomicrograph illustrating the simple columnar epithelium (arrows), lamina propria (LP), and intertwining of circular (C) and longitudinal (L) smooth muscle of the muscularis of the oviduct. × 140.

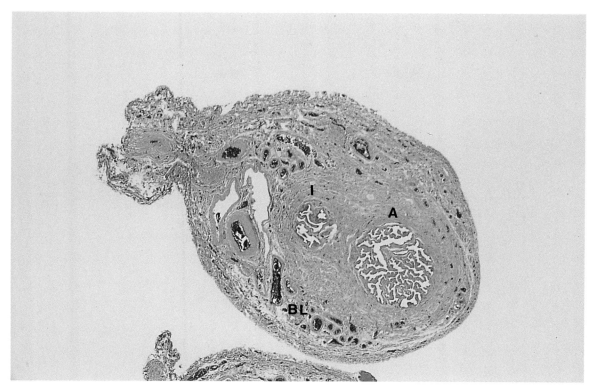

figure 19-15

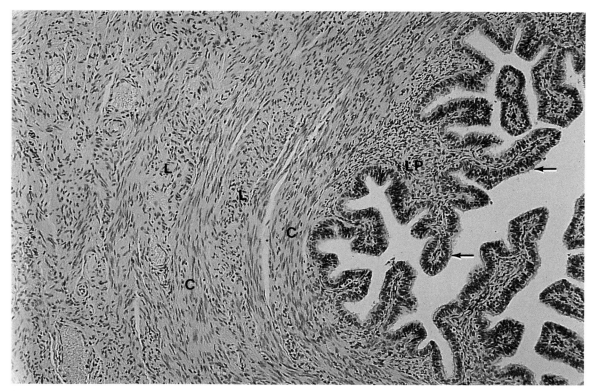

figure 19-16

FIGURE 19-17
Photomicrograph illustrating the endometrium (E) and myometrium (M) of the uterus. L, lumen. × 14.

FIGURE 19-18
Photomicrograph showing the stratum basalis (B) of the endometrium and a portion of the myometrium (M) of the uterus. × 56.

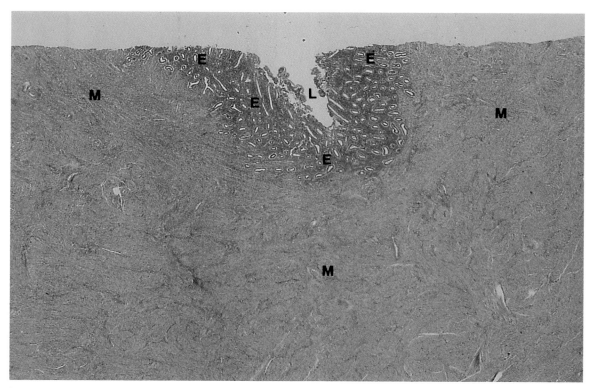

figure 19-17

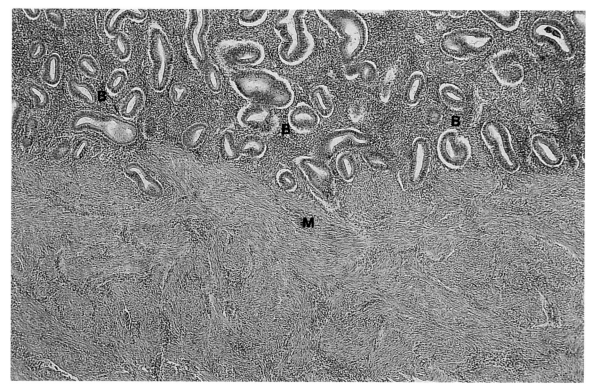

figure 19-18

FIGURE 19-22
Photomicrograph of a portion of the uterine cervix. At the junction (J) of the endocervical
(EC) and vaginal (V) parts of the cervix, the cervical epithelium abruptly changes from
simple columnar (SC) to stratified squamous (SS). Note the cervical glands (unlabeled
arrows). V, vagina. × 14.

FIGURE 19-23
Photomicrograph illustrating the stratified squamous epithelium (E), lamina propria (L),
lamina muscularis (M), and fibroelastic connective tissue of the vagina. Note the lym-
phocytic infiltration (arrows) in the lamina propria. × 56.

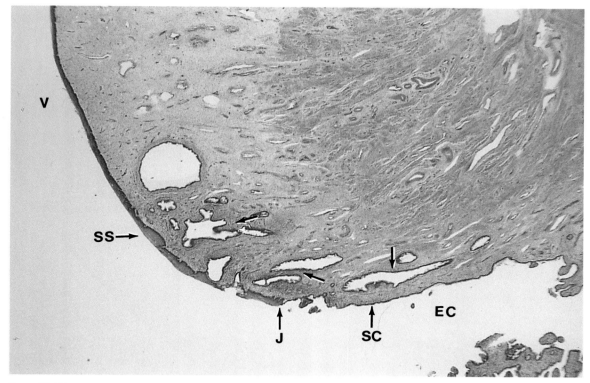

figure 19-22

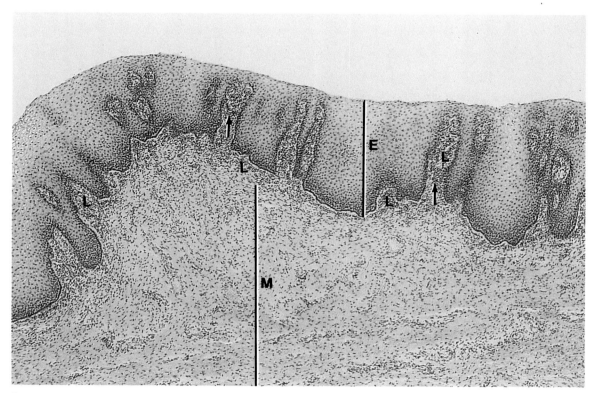

figure 19-23

FIGURE 19-24
Photomicrograph of a section of an inactive mammary gland. The glandular tissue within the lobules (L) is not well developed and is composed primarily of duct elements. Note the abundant interlobular connective tissue (CT). × 56.

FIGURE 19-25
Photomicrograph of an active but nonlactating mammary gland. The glandular elements of lobules (L) are much more highly developed than those in Figure 19-24. Note the ducts (D) in the much reduced dense irregular interlobular connective tissue (CT). A, adipose tissue. × 56.

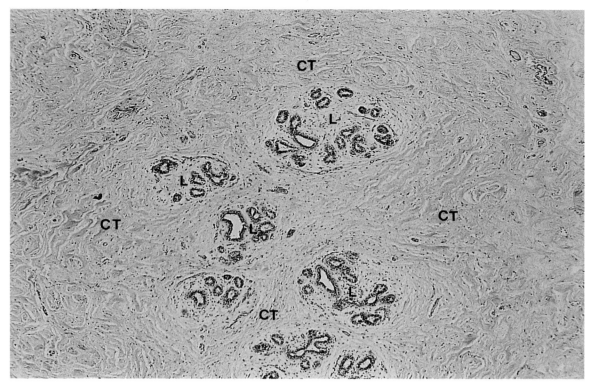

figure 19-24

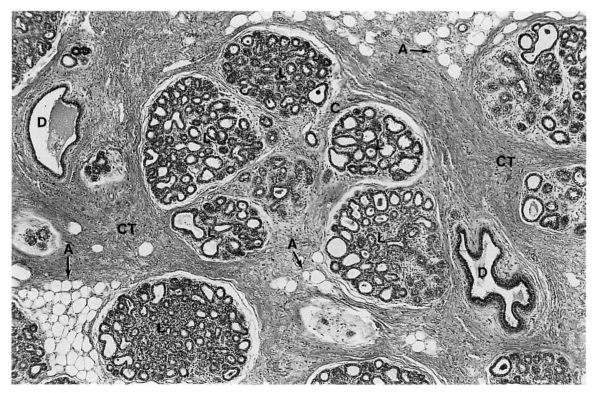

figure 19-25

FIGURE 19-26
Photomicrograph of a lactating mammary gland. Note the paucity of interlobular connective tissue (arrows); note also the alveoli (A) and ducts (D) with milk. Compare with Figures 19-24 and 19-25. × 56.

FIGURE 19-27
Photomicrograph of ducts (D) and alveoli (A) from a lobule of an active but nonlactating mammary gland. Note the stratified cuboidal epithelium of the ducts and simple cuboidal epithelium of the alveoli. A plasma cell (P), lymphocytes (L), fibroblasts (F), milk (unlabeled arrows), and a blood vessel (V) are also seen in the loose irregular intralobular connective tissue. CT, interlobular connective tissue. × 344.

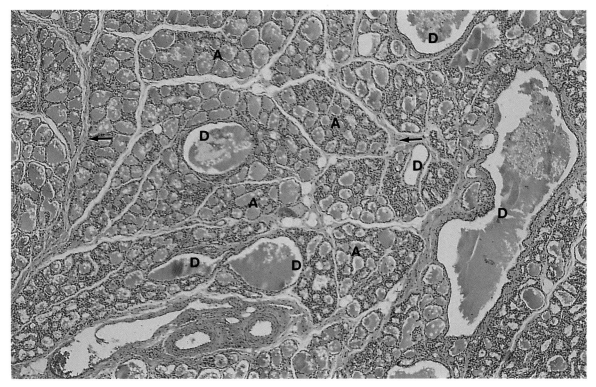

figure 19-26

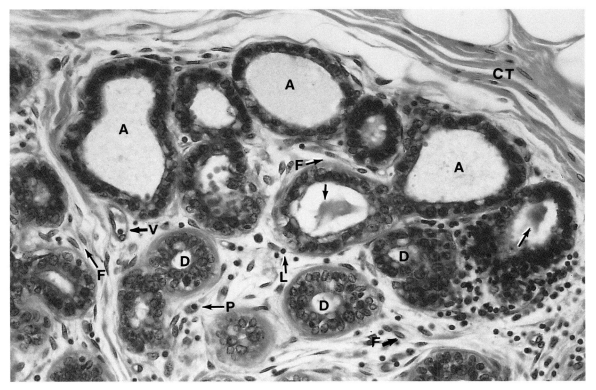

figure 19-27

20 The Sense Organs

FIGURE 20-1

Photomicrograph of the anterior portion of the eye illustrating the cornea (C), anterior chamber (AC), iris (i), lens (L), the major substance of which was extracted during slide preparation, ciliary body (CB), and conjunctiva (CO). Monkey; × 14.

FIGURE 20-2

Photomicrograph of the cornea of the eye illustrating epithelium (E), stroma (S), Descemet's membrane (d), and endothelium (En). Monkey; × 140.

FIGURE 20-3

Photomicrograph of the optic nerve (ON) from the eye adjacent to the optic papilla. Bar, neural and pigmented retina; BV, blood vessels. Monkey; × 56.

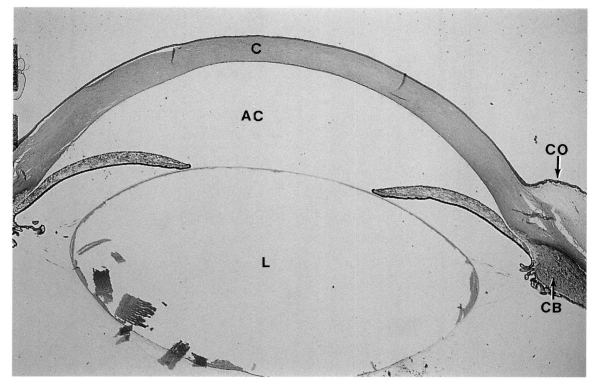

figure 20-1

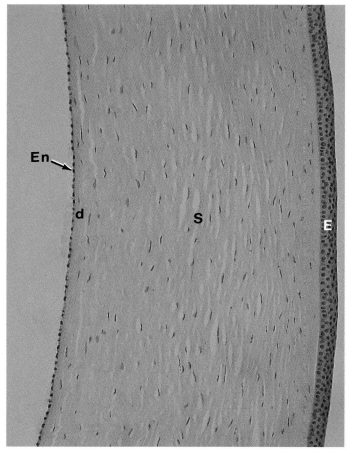

figure 20-2

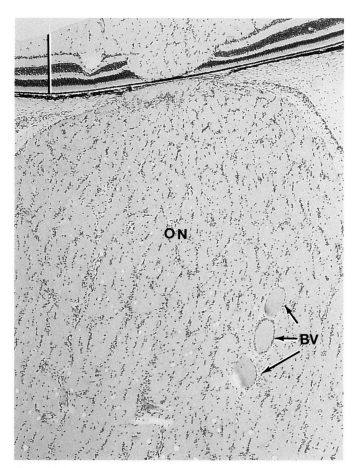

figure 20-3

FIGURE 20-4

Photomicrograph of the iris of the eye illustrating the stoma (S), constrictor pupillae muscle (CP), dilator pupillae muscle (DP), pigmented epithelium (PE), anterior (AC) and posterior (PC) chambers of the eye, and a portion of the lens (L), the major substance of which was extracted during slide preparation. Monkey; × 140.

FIGURE 20-5

Photomicrograph of the ciliary body of the eye illustrating the smooth muscle of the ciliary body (SM), ciliary processes (C), epithelium of the ciliary processes (E), pigmented epithelium of the iris (PE), and suspensory ligament (SL). Monkey; × 140.

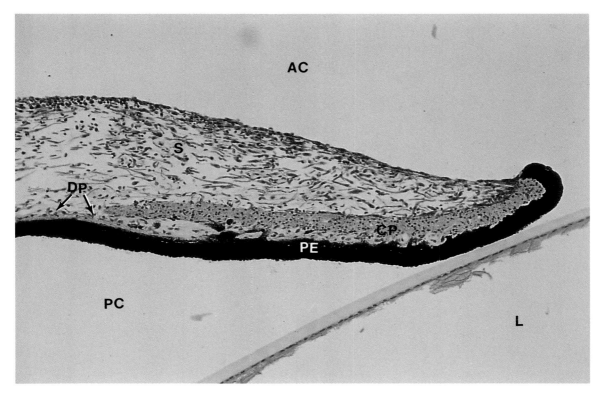

figure 20-4

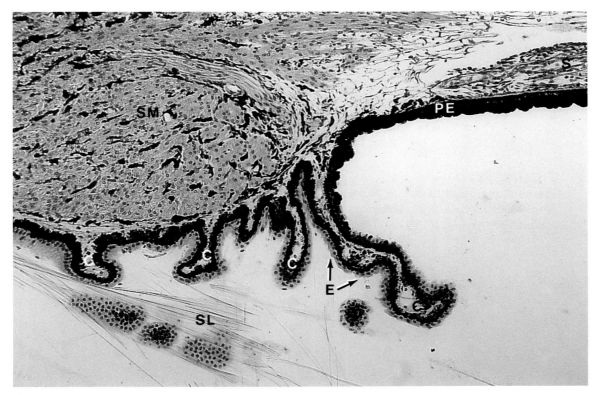

figure 20-5

FIGURE 20-6
Photomicrograph of part of the ciliary body and iris of the eye illustrating the smooth muscle of the ciliary body (SM), trabecular meshwork of the corneoscleral junction (T), canal of Schlemm (CS), anterior chamber (AC), stroma of the iris (S), and pigmented epithelium of the iris (PE). Monkey; × 140.

FIGURE 20-7
Photomicrograph illustrating the canal of Schlemm (CS), trabecular meshwork of the corneoscleral junction (T), anterior chamber (AC), stroma of the iris (S), and pigmented epithelium of the iris (PE) of the eye. Monkey; × 344.

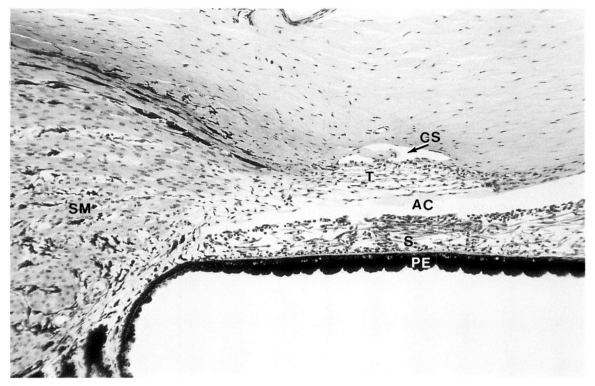

figure 20-6

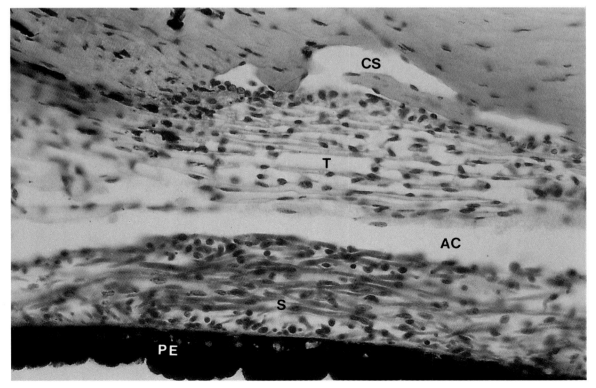

figure 20-7

FIGURE 20-8
Photomicrograph of the wall of the eye illustrating the retina (bar), choroid (C), sclera
(S), and periorbital adipose tissue (P). Monkey; × 56.

FIGURE 20-9
Photomicrograph of the sensory (neural) and pigmented parts of the retina of the eye.
Shown are the inner limiting membrane (1), ganglion cell fiber layer (2), ganglion cell
layer (3), inner plexiform layer (4), inner nuclear layer (5), outer plexiform layer (6), outer
nuclear layer (7), outer limiting membrane (8), rods and cones (9), and pigmented layer
(10). C, choroid. Monkey; × 140.

FIGURE 20-10
Higher-power photomicrograph of the outer part of the retina of the eye depicted in
Figure 20-9. Shown are the outer plexiform layer (6), outer nuclear layer (7), outer
limiting membrane (8), inner segment (IS) and outer segment (OS) of the rods and cones
(9), and pigmented cell layer (10). Monkey; × 869.

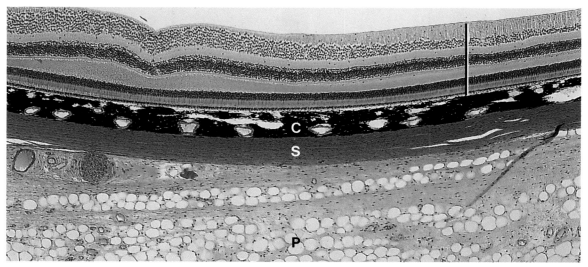

figure 20-8

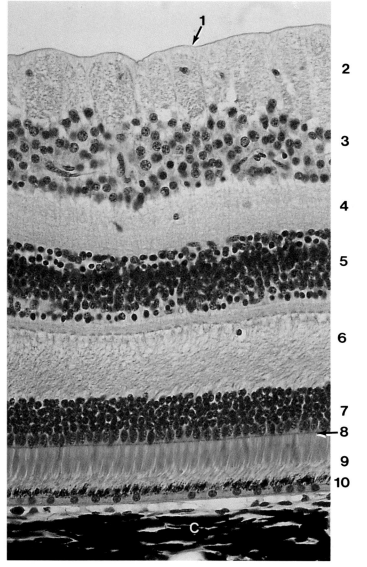

figure 20-9

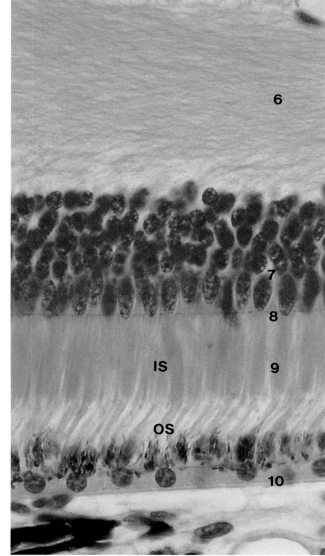

figure 20-10

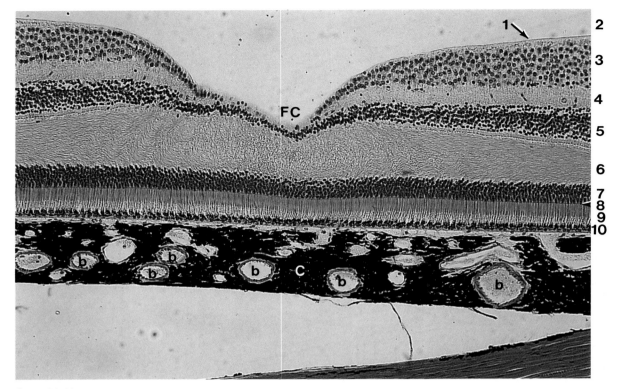

figure 20-11

FIGURE 20-11
Photomicrograph of the fovea centralis (FC) of the eye. Note the numerous blood vessels (b) in the choroid (C). Refer to Figure 20-9 for the layers of the retina. Monkey; × 56.

FIGURE 20-12
Photomicrograph illustrating olfactory and respiratory mucosae. Note the absence of goblet cells in olfactory epithelium (OE), in contrast to numerous goblet cells (unlabeled arrows) in the respiratory epithelium (RE). B, bone. Monkey; × 56.

FIGURE 20-13
Photomicrograph of olfactory mucosa. Note the sustentacular (SC), olfactory (OC), and basal (BC) cells of the olfactory epithelium. LP, lamina propria; G, glands; B, bone; V, blood vessel. Monkey; × 144.

FIGURE 20-14
Higher-power photomicrograph of part of the olfactory mucosa depicted in Figure 20-13. SC, sustentacular cells; OC, olfactory cells; arrows, basal cells; G, glands; N, nerve bundle; B, bone. Monkey; × 344.

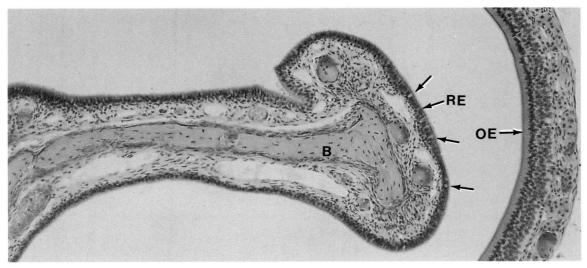

figure 20-12

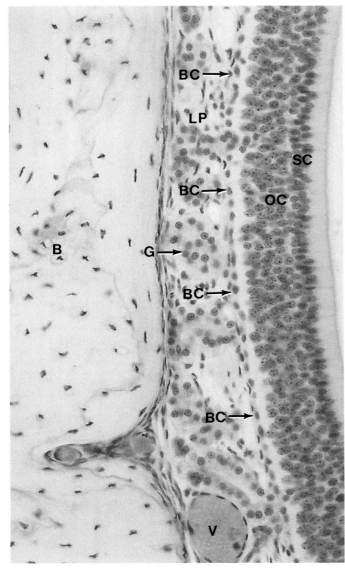

figure 20-13

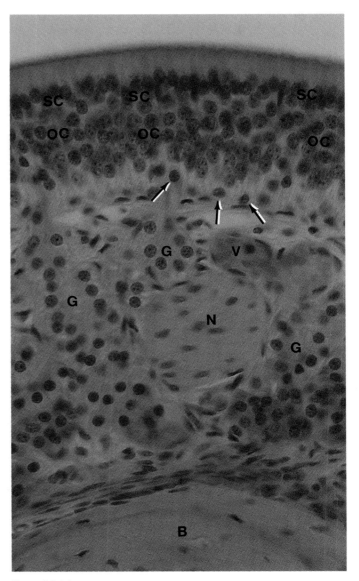

figure 20-14

FIGURE 20-15
Survey micrograph of the internal ear illustrating the helicotrema (H), spiral ganglion (G), scala vestibula (SV), cochlear duct (CD), scala tympani (ST), cochlear nerve (CN), modiolus (M), vestibule (V), stapes (S), ducts of the membranous labyrinth (Dm), bone (B), and facial nerve (FN). Guinea pig; × 14.

FIGURE 20-16
Higher-power photomicrograph of part of Figure 20-15 illustrating the helicotrema (H), organ of Corti (OC), spiral ganglion (G), scala vestibula (SV), vestibular membrane (VM), cochlear duct (CD), scala tympani (ST), cochlear nerve (CN), and bone (B). Guinea pig; × 56.

FIGURE 20-17
Photomicrograph of part of the spiral ganglion (G) of the internal ear. N, nerve bundles; B, bone. Guinea pig; × 344.

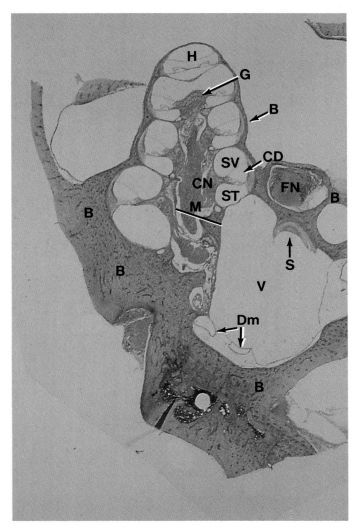

figure 20-15

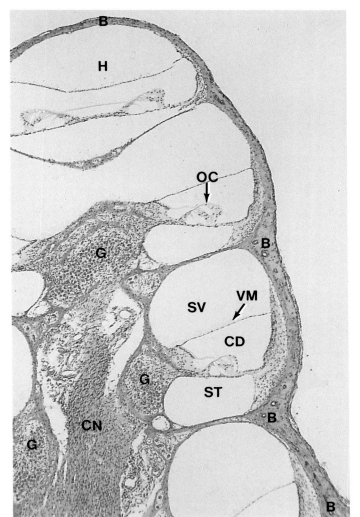

figure 20-16

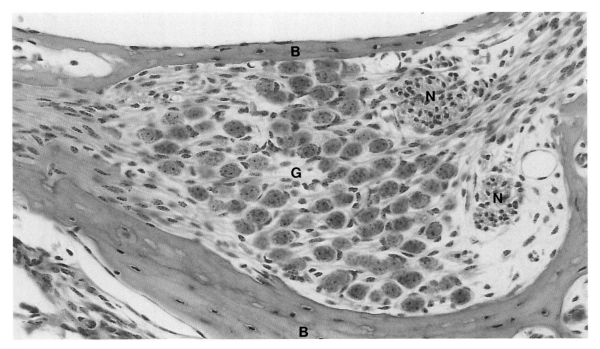

figure 20-17

FIGURE 20-18
Photomicrograph of part of the cochlea of the internal ear illustrating the organ of Corti (OC), tectoral membrane (Tm), cochlear duct (CD), stria vascularis (StV), vestibular membrane (Vm), scala vestibula (SV), spiral ligament (SL), scala tympani (ST), cochlear nerve (CN), limbus spiralis (LS), osseous spiral lamina (OSL), spiral ganglion (G), and bone (B). Guinea pig; × 140.

FIGURE 20-19
Photomicrograph illustrating the components of the organ of Corti. This photomicrograph is oriented 90° differently from that in Figure 20-18. Shown are the inner phalangeal cells (IP), inner hair cell (IHC), inner pilar cells (IPC), inner tunnel (IT), outer pilar cell (OPC), outer phalangeal cell (OP), outer hair cell (OHC), outer tunnel (OT), outer border cells (OBC), inner spiral tunnel (IST), inner border cells (IBC), limbus spiralis (LS), osseous spiral lamina (OSL), cochlear nerve (CN), vestibular membrane (Vm), tectoral membrane (Tm), and basement membrane (Bm). Guinea pig; × 344.

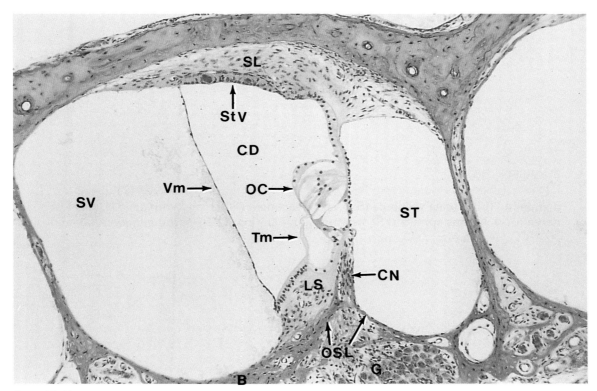

figure 20-18

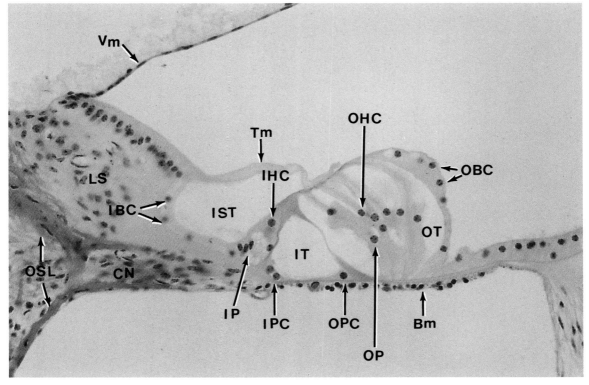

figure 20-19

FIGURE 20-20
Photomicrograph of foliate papillae (which are not prominent in human tongue) showing taste buds (unlabeled arrows). E, stratified squamous epithelium; CT, connective tissue; V, von Ebner's glands; D, ducts of von Ebner's glands; S, skeletal muscle. Rabbit; × 140.

FIGURE 20-21
Higher-power photomicrograph of the lateral surfaces of foliate papillae. Note the taste buds (unlabeled arrows), pores (P) of the taste buds, and stratified squamous epithelium (E) of the papillae. Rabbit; × 560.

FIGURE 20-22
Photomicrograph of two taste buds showing dark cells (DC), light cells (LC), and basal cells (BC). Note the taste bud pores (P). Rabbit; × 869.

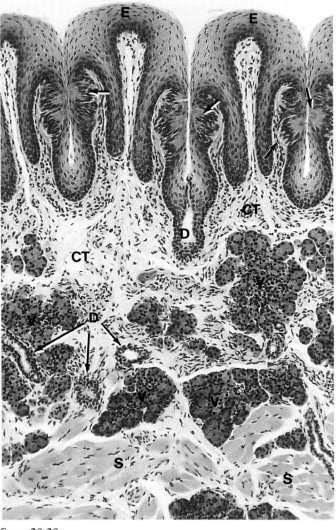

figure 20-20

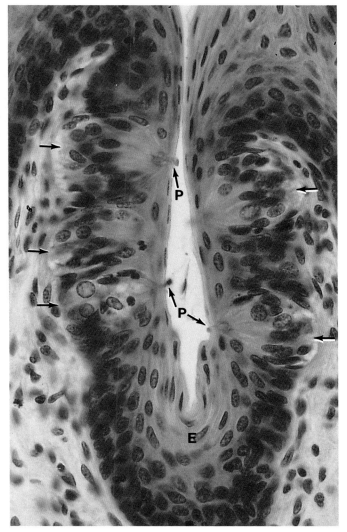

figure 20-21

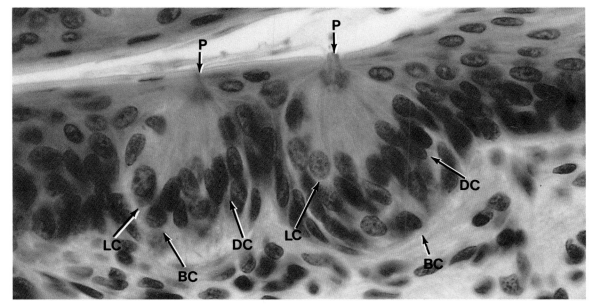

figure 20-22

Index

Entries correspond to figure numbers except when page numbers are denoted by *italics*.